Structured
Water

for Greater Health
and Happiness

Michael D. Miller

Copyright 2009

1

Table of Contents

Here is a quick history about structured water:

In a Nutshell:

In Austria, back in the 1930s, a young forest warden by the name of Viktor Shauberger made some startling observations. He noticed that trout in a fast moving mountain stream were able to dart about at fast speeds that could not be explained by the movement of their fins alone. He concluded that the tumbling and spinning of the fast moving mountain streams imparted an energy to the fish that allowed for their fast movement. Using this knowledge, he became famous for his ability to manipulate water for large successful water projects. He also demonstrated that water energized by tumbling and spinning down a mountain stream had distinctive health benefits. Crops grew better and animals and people were healthier when they drank this water.

When Germany took over Austria, Shauberger was forced by the Nazis to set up a laboratory to further his developments. He made some amazing scientific discoveries about the ability of "structured" water to generate energy and power.

At the end of WWII the American Army forcibly placed Shauberger in a remote military base in South Texas where they replicated his experiments. He remained there until just before he died ten years later. His discoveries about the structure of water have never been made public. However a fascinating book, "Living

Energies" by Callum Coates is available on amazon.com and it finally reveals much about this fascinating man and his work to structure water to benefit mankind.

In the 1980s a chemist, Jim Sheridan, working for the Dow Chemical Company in Midland, Michigan, decided to seek a chemical cure for cancer. Working alone, and on his spare time, he made considerable progress. But he was consistently thwarted by his inability to get governmental approvals for his work. Eventually he brought in another friend to assist him named Ed Sopcak. Ed was an electrical engineer. Unable to make Jim's method work, Ed undertook another approach. He sought an electrical approach. Eventually he was successful, and they developed a liquid that they called Cancell.

To avoid problems with the government, they decided to give their healing liquid away for free. They set up a separate telephone line to receive orders. I attempted to place an order as soon as I heard about this. But the line was always busy. Apparently business was good! Eventually I got through, and they dutifully sent me my free clear liquid remedy.

But disaster struck. Even though they were giving their remedy away for free, the government shut them down. Lest you doubt my story, a book on amazon.com, "The Cancell Controversy" by Louise B. Trull tells the whole story. Several years later Ed Sopcak , although less than fifty years old, died somewhat mysteriously. So it appeared that his discovery had died with him.

But not so. Researchers established that he had removed the memory form water and then imparted energies of love and healing to the water. Thus this positively energized water interrupted the negative energy patterns of disease, disabling it so that the body's own immune system could eradicate the disease.

Say what? Water has memory? This is esoteric stuff. Never heard that before. And the knowledge died with Ed Sopcak.

But not so.

Ten years later a Japanese scientist by the name of Masaru Emoto made an amazing discovery. He flash froze water molecules. He then photographed each water molecule as it went from the liquid state to the solid state. He also experimented. He found that when he spoke to the freezing water molecule, it affected the shape of the molecule. If he said positive things, such as "I love you" to the water molecule, it transformed into a beautiful white crystalline shape, similar to that of a snowflake. If he spoke harshly, saying "I hate you", the water molecule shriveled and became dark. Dr. Emoto was rediscovering that water does hold memory and appears to have a consciousness. Weird stuff.

He wrote a book about his discovery, complete with pictures, and it became a New York Time's bestseller! "The Hidden Messages in Water", available on amazon.com, became a worldwide sensation. There is also much information on the Internet about this structured water discovery.

So I now knew more about Ed Sopcak's discovery. But I did not know how to reprogram water to make it a healing agent. Years went by. Then I attended several summer conferences of the Tesla Society. Following the discoveries and inventions of Nikola Tesla, these yearly conferences are attended by hundreds of interesting "backyard" inventors and scientists. These guys really think outside the box! So I approached them for help. Within a few hours I had my answers. These wonderful minds freely exchange information, and they helped me immensely.

Now I know how to make structured water that heals and structured water that energizes.

But this information would not be complete without knowledge of Ormus Water. In the 1980s a wealthy Arizona cotton farmer and experimenter named David Hudson made some interesting discoveries, finding an atomic substance that appeared unknown to mankind. After several million dollars of research, it was realized that he had rediscovered the substance previously known in other ages as the Philosopher Stone. Manna, and the elixir of life. In structured water it is a healing and rejuvenating agent. We have, after years of experimentation and research, learned how to make this ormus structured water cheaply and easily. This is information that you do not want to miss out on.

I also have found a company that makes a healing herbal tea, and they make it with structured water that uses the principles that are detailed in this handbook.. How clever. Kind of like killing two birds with one stone. The herbal tea heals and the water it is made from heals. See http://www.remedies.net for more information.

w let's get going. The first section we will devote to Ormus water. I especially suggest that you note the sacred geometry method of making ormus water. This is the method that I use. I drink 4 glasses of this water each day, and it appears to be working.

Section A: The Ormus story

An amazing rejuvenation method for longevity

Our Anti-Aging and Health Secret

This is just may be the most important information that you will ever read. Does this sound hard to believe? Just wait and see! This information is not for people who have are faint of heart, nor is it for the person who cannot think outside of the box. But this info is for people who really want to be young for as long as possible. It is for the open-minded person who is willing to concede that there are still some secrets to anti aging and eternal beauty that are out there and still are to be discovered.

It took special people to once consider that perhaps the world was not flat, perhaps man could fly, perhaps there was a cure for polio. Now we ask you to consider that perhaps there is a way to reverse the aging process, perhaps there is a way to restore health and vigor, to make people younger, and to reverse the aging process.

I know how many of you feel right now. Shock, disbelief and skepticism have set in. But please bear with me. I don't ask for you to believe me. **I do ask that you keep an open mind**; I do ask that you listen now to what I have to say. Should you not believe me, you can always discard this information later. But if you do not listen to my message, you do not have the opportunity to benefit, to learn how to regain your youth and health, how to reverse the aging process, and how to get the sharp, focused and alert mind that you had as a young person.

For you see, this is information was rediscovered about twenty years ago, but its use to maintain vigor and youthfulness is still pretty much unknown. So if you are an older person who wants to be youthful for many more years, please give us a chance to explain things to you.

We say that this anti-aging information was "rediscovered" because the ancients knew this information. A study of the ancient religions of India, Tibet, Egypt, and Israel reveals fascinating evidence that this anti-aging knowledge was possessed by them. Then, during the middle ages, this knowledge was passed on to European sources. At various times it was referred to as manna (the bible), shewbread (The ancient Egyptians), and the Philosopher Stone (the middle ages). Sound wild? Are you brave enough to stick with us? We will discuss this more in a minute.

The concept that a secret substance can be produced from certain metals (gold, silver, platinum, rhodium and iridium) that is capable of expanding consciousness, extending longevity, and enhancing health, is hard to grasp. It is hard to accept. It challenges our most basic belief systems. I know, because I have been where you are right now. Please stick with me for a while longer. I stuck it out, and I am now certainly glad that I did. I sincerely hope that you will stick it out.

What we have to offer you is not difficult or expensive to try out. So what have you got to lose?

Originally, as practiced by the ancients in the Far East and the Middle East, this mystical material that they had learned to extract from gold was used strictly for spiritual enlightenment and rejuvenation. But later, when this information was transferred to Europe, the emphasis was changed to using the material, now known as "The Philosopher Stone", to transmute lead into gold.

A Historical Perspective

Right now I am struggling as to how to convince you that this information is true and valid. Let's begin by looking at some ancient historical references to our white powder of gold.

So I will jump to something that we all know about, the bible. Sometimes great truths are hidden right out in the open.

The Bible Speaks of It.

The old testament talks about how, during the Exodus, Moses went up into the mountains to pray for 40 days. See Exodus, Chapter 32; 1-35. When Moses came down, he found that the people had made a golden calf and they were worshipping the golden calf. The bible says that an angry Moses seized the golden calf and burned it, and he then fed the burnt gold to the people. Also, later, during their sojourn through the deserts, the bible says that Moses fed the people a substance that they called "manna", and it sustained them during their time of travail.

This story of Moses, told to me since I was a child, never made sense. You do not burn gold, you melt it. And you cannot feed molten gold to anybody. But, as did everyone else, I never sought to question the bible.

Now, after the years that I have spent researching this subject, I know that Moses had been raised by the Pharaoh's daughter and had access to many of the teachings of the high-ranking Egyptian priests. He had learned their secret of processing gold to extract a white powder that was a powdered monatomic form of gold. This white powder of gold was assimilated by people, and it renewed their DNA in order to reestablish their youthful health and vigor.

It is believed that Moses learned from the Priests that this knowledge of how to make the white powder of gold (that they baked into small loaves known as shewbread) had been given them by the Atlanteans who colonized Egypt some 5,000 years previously.

The Far East

I have in my possession a copy of an ancient Hindu text. It was written by an Indian scholar. This text explains the ancient Indian practice and knowledge of transmuting base metal into gold. Over twenty very exact formulas, as practiced by Indian sages several hundred years ago, for making gold are presented. All of these formulas involve using a base metal (mercury or lead), mixing it with a form of fresh mashed herbs or plants, and performing prayerful ceremonies over the process for some thirty days. The formulas are all very specific that the proper prayerful intent must be present for such processes to proceed. They also stress that only the "pure of heart" will be successful.

This text tells some interesting, if also a bit tragic, stories. It seems that when the British subjugated India, the British authorities learned of certain spiritual gurus who with certain regularity materialized gold. These gurus were forthwith arrested and interrogated to extract their secrets. Under severe interrogation (including torture), some 57 spiritual gurus were forced to reveal their formulas. They, for the most part, and given the circumstances, were willing to give away this knowledge.

When the British authorities tried these formulas, they failed. The gurus had known that this would happen because of the impurity of the British experimenters. Frustrated, and believing that the gurus had withheld necessary information, the British further tortured the gurus. But there was nothing that the gurus could do; without a certain purity of heart and intention on the part of the British people conducting the transmutation process, it could not be successful. All of the gurus died.

Meanwhile there was a prominent guru who had avoided arrest. He knew the secrets. He wished to protest the deaths of his compatriots. He announced to the people that at a certain time on a certain day he would appear at the main gate of the prominent city of Madras. He had a message for the British.

He appeared at the main gate of the city, as promised. He extracted a small cloth bag from his garments. He took an amount of a powdered substance from the cloth bag. He slowly rubbed the powder onto one of the massive iron gates. After a few minutes the heavy, 10 foot tall iron gate suddenly transmuted into gold. The guru quickly disappeared.

This guru had made his point, reminding the British authorities that their lack of purity would mean that they could never replicate what the pure-of-spirit-gurus could do. The British took this massive metal (now gold) gate down, and they shipped it to London where it is believed to still reside deep in the bowels of a British museum.

By the way, the ancient alchemists of Europe were also adamant that a pure heart and purity of intent was a necessary qualification of any alchemist who would attempt to transmute mercury or lead into gold.

One in-depth study of the alchemical tradition of India is told by David Gordon White in his book "The Alchemical Body". He tells of the widespread use of alchemy by the spiritual leaders of India in the first millennium AD. Then there is the Rig Veda, the ancient Hindu text that extensively discusses the "food of the gods" that is derived from gold. It was believed to be written during the period from 4000BC to 11,000BC. These, as well as many other references, establish that alchemy was a prominent part of the spiritual practices of ancient India.

Europe

Some scholars will tell you that all of this is balderdash. They insist that this is all a fabricated hoax, and that mankind has never known how to make gold out of other metals. Here I have an interesting bit of information. It is a historical fact that at various times in the past, the governments of Europe passed laws forbidding the manufacture (transmutation) of gold. So I pose the question: If mankind never knew how to make gold, why outlaw it? I await an answer.

In 1317 the new pope, John XXII, issued a decree banning the alchemical production of gold. In 1380 King Charles V also banned using alchemy to make gold.

It is believed that outlawing the manufacture (transmutation) of gold was done for several purposes. First of all, too much gold introduced into the marketplace would have the effect of debasing the established currency. Second, in several instances, the governmental leaders had learned the secrets of alchemical transformation of gold, and they wished to eliminate the competition. Very clever. In one instance, King Henry IV of England coerced an alchemist into revealing his secret process for making gold. Then, after the king had successfully mastered this secret process, the king had the alchemist jailed for life, and then the king passed a law forbidding the alchemical transformation of base metals into gold. King Henry thus had an exclusive!

Also, the Inquisition caused much havoc amongst the alchemists of Europe. Finding themselves very vulnerable to charges of heresy and "witchery", the alchemists of Europe went underground for many hundreds of years. What few writings of theirs that have survived are of dubious value because their knowledges are so carefully disguised and camouflaged in obtuse writing that it is almost impossible to decipher them.

In France the alchemist Nicholas Flamel was famous for his alchemical knowledge. His works are still studied today, and his residence (in a prominent neighborhood on the left bank) in Paris is now a museum. It was widely known that he made gold. But he was very clever. Although no one could explain where his evident prosperity came from, neither could they ever catch him making gold.

Likewise the person known as Saint Germaine was widely known to transmute base metals into gold. St. Germaine was a friend and confidante to the kings and queens of Europe. He lived extravagantly, always travelling and living in the manner of the royalty. He, too, was clever and his secrets were never revealed.

In this book we will give you the overview of what we have discovered. This book will tell you everything that you need to reverse the aging process and regain full and total health.

But some of you will wish to research this fascinating subject more deeply. For those people, we will also provide a bibliography of the relevant texts that you may wish to verify what we have told you, or to seek greater details of what we are about to tell you

How and Why We Age

There you have it. This is our anti aging secret.

But to understand our secret completely, you have to know how a person ages. Our bodies are made up of millions of cells. Each cell has a life of about seven years. So, every seven years or so, each cell in our body is replaced by a new cell. Within each cell is something that we know as DNA. This DNA is the blueprint for that cell. So when it is time for a new cell to form, the DNA strand within the old cell tells the new cell how to grow. It, in effect, is the blueprint for what the new cell is supposed to look like. So, using this blueprint, the new cell grows up and replaces the dying cell. When you are a young person, the older cell in your body is still in good shape, and its DNA blueprint of what it should be is still very accurate. So the blueprint that it shows to the new growing replacement cell is very accurate, and this the new cell will grow up to look like, and be just like the older cell. Thus people continue to look young and attractive, as their bodies are continually replenished with cells that are young and vibrant.

But as we age things change. A mature person's situation is not the same. Hers or his body has, over the years, been subjected to the harshness of life. Each person has been subjected to the stresses of life. People are also bombarded constantly with toxins in the food, and in the air we breathe. Lack of sufficient rest and relaxation also take a toll. As does emotional weariness. All of these elements tend to damage the DNA strand that is in each cell of each person's body.

Thus it is that older people's bodies are different that the bodies of younger people. For when it is time for an aging cell in an older mature person's body to be replaced, the blueprint that the newly forming cell will need to use as a guide as to what it should look and be like has been damaged. Damaged by accumulated toxins and poisons, emotional stress and exhaustion, the older person's DNA gives a less-than-perfect blueprint of what the new cell should like. Thus the new cell is not quite like the cell that it has replaced. It is less vibrant and healthy. Thus aging sets in.

This, in short, is why men and women age.

The Modern Discovery

So how does this relate to the information that I desire to pass along to you? Well, what mankind discovered long ago, back in ancient times, has been rediscovered. It has been rediscovered that there is a special form of substance that is extracted from certain precious metals (mostly gold) and certain types of sea water. This substance performs the function of renewing and rebuilding the damaged strands of DNA in an older man or woman.

In 1988 a wealthy Arizona cotton farmer by the name of David Hudson set out to analyze the soils on some of his cotton farms. He knew that the Spaniards had mined gold on these lands, and he sought to find out if there were any remaining precious metal deposits. So he sent samples of his soils in to laboratories for analysis. In the resulting chemical and spectrographic analysis, a substance was discovered that did not to seem to fit into the modern table of elements. After much further study, it was determined that they had stumbled upon a yet-as-unknown substance. Eventually he realized that he had rediscovered the material that had been known by the ancients for its ability to restore youthfulness and vitality.

David Hudson's full and amazing story is too long to repeat here. But if you choose to "google" on "David Hudson", or "Ormus" or "Ormes", or "White powder of gold" a whole new world of anti aging information will open up to you.

I have spent years researching this subject. I have, over the years, experimented with making certain forms of the element. I have been taking one form or another of the substance for some ten years now. I am sixty-nine years old. I have watched in amazement as my gray hair turned black again, and how the lines and wrinkles in my face have disappeared. I also wonder at the way my memory has improved, and how I now realize that my mind is as sharp as it ever was, maybe even sharper. I relish in showing people a photo that was taken of me when I was 57 years old (twelve years ago), and compare it with a photo that was taken last year. I look younger and healthier in the photo that was taken last year.

But how do you tell people of something that is so unbelievable? I have tried many times. It is difficult. It is discouraging. And I don't particularly blame the people who give me a blank stare and walk off. It does seem unbelievable.

But then I am reminded of the story of penicillin, the first antibiotic. Penicillin was first discovered in 1893. But nobody would try it because it seemed too unbelievable. It was too good to be true. For fifty years no one would try it. Then in 1943, during the medical emergencies of WWII, out of desperation it was tried. It worked! And it, and the other antibiotic medicines that have followed, have changed our lived dramatically.

Well, the open-minded people who read this blurb may just well be like the first brave souls who tried penicillin. These people will be trendsetters. They will be pioneers along with the few others of us who have taken advantage of this wonderful anti aging discovery.

And thank you for listening to my story. If you have gotten to this part of my write-up, I am sure that you are a brave and open-minded person.

The David Hudson Story as he tells it:

This is part of a transcript of a February 1995 introductory lecture and workshop by David Hudson in Dallas, Texas. It was transcribed from the video tapes which were recorded on February 10 and 11, 1995. The video tapes are available from The Eclectic Viewpoint, P.O. Box 802735, Dallas, Texas 75380. Contact hot line (214) 601-7687.

The video tapes have readable pictures of all of the documents that Hudson references. The serious student of these subjects will find these tapes are worth obtaining. The package of three video tapes costs $69.95 plus $5.00 for shipping and handling.

[**David Hudson speaks**] "Basically this is the story of my quest for this material. I wanted to get an understanding of it, to be able to explain what it is. And my work began in this area for all the wrong reasons. I did not understand what I was doing. I didn't understand what the material was and it's only in the last four or five years that I've really come to an understanding, understanding truly of what the material really is. But basically the work began about 1975-76, and my primary interest for getting into this area is, was, like I say, for all the wrong reasons.

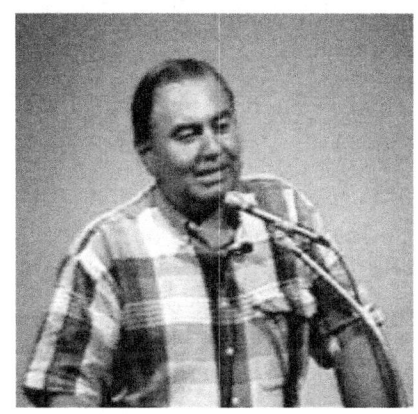

I am from Phoenix, Arizona. My father is the ex-commissioner of agriculture in the state of Arizona. My mother is the, was the state Republican's woman chairman. We're ultra-ultra right-wing conservative. Very, very ultra conservative people. All of my farming was done on a handshake basis. I even farmed 2,500 acres on a handshake with the Bureau of Indian Affairs and that's the federal government and no one farms with the federal government on a handshake and a verbal agreement but I did.

Our family is very, very conservative, very highly regarded in the community. All my vehicles have the keys in the vehicles right now. I'm here and they're there. Ah, we just... it's a very small community just outside of Phoenix where, you know, everyone knows everybody. Everybody

19

knows the people going down the road. There just is no theft.

Anyway, when I became involved in this my thinking was to mine and process gold and silver to keep for myself. I was very disillusioned with the federal government's approach to our currency. They were devaluing the dollar, issuing this funny money, what they called Federal Reserve notes which I'm sure most of you people are aware of. They were not backed by gold and silver, and as you make more and more of these dollars they continue to devalue these dollars and you think you are making more money, but in fact all you are doing is moving into a higher tax bracket and paying more and more income tax. And so you have less and less even though you are making more and more.

Anyway, I began buying gold and silver in the Phoenix area as bullion from refiners. Most of it was being refined from sterling silver scrap or electronic scrap. But, ah, a lot of the gold was coming from miners who were processing it by a process called "heap leach cyanide recovery". And they were heap leaching, um, these old tailings on these mining operations. I became very intrigued with this because we were very interested, in agriculture, in metal salts in our soils. I don't know, I think that here in Dallas it's much the same or further on west in the state, it's much the same as Arizona. We have a sodium problem in our soil. It's called "black alkali" and as the black alkali builds up in your soil you can put sulfuric acid on the soil and the sodium, which makes up the black alkali, becomes sodium sulfate, which is a white alkali. And then is water soluble and will leach out of your soil then. If you don't do this your soil is very oily and the water just won't penetrate and be retained by the soil and it's not very good for your crops.

And so we had been doing soils analysis and this concept of, of literally piling ore up on a piece of plastic and spraying it with a cyanide solution, which dissolves selectively the gold out of the ore. It trickles down through the ore until it hits the plastic and then runs out the plastic and into the settling pond. It's pumped up through activated charcoal where the gold adheres to the charcoal and then the solution is returned back to the stack. And the concept seemed pretty simple, and I decided, you know, a lot of farmers have airplanes, a lot of farmers have race horses, a lot of farmers have race cars... I decided I was going to have a gold mine. And, I had earth movers and water trucks and road graders and backhoes and caterpillars and these kinds of things on the farm and I had equipment operators, and so I decided I was going to set up one of these heap leach cyanide systems.

I traveled all over the state of Arizona, took about a year and a half, and I finally settled on a piece of property. And, ah, did some analysis and all and decided that this was the property that had the gold in it that I wanted to recover. I set up a heap leach cyanide system, began spraying the ore, and sure enough within a matter of a couple days, we hooked it up to the activated charcoal. And we analyzed the solution going in the charcoal. We analyzed the solution coming out of the charcoal and we were loading gold on the charcoal. And, you know, everything is just rosy. We're having a high old time. And I figured I could lose 50 percent per year mining gold and be as well off as buying the gold and paying taxes at 50 percent on the, on the profit with buying the gold. So, if other people had to mine gold and make a living, I could mine gold and lose 50 percent, and be as well off as making the money, paying income tax and buying gold with it. So I figured, hey, I ought to be able to do that.

21

So, what happened is, ah, we began recovering the gold and silver and we would take the charcoal down to our farm. We'd strip it with hot cyanide and sodium hydroxide. We'd run it through "electro winning cell". We'd get the gold out on the "electro winning cell". And then we would do what's called a "fire assay" where you run it through a crucible reduction. Now I am not going to elaborate on all this because I am not trying to teach anybody "fire assaying". I am just trying to explain the procedures here. This is the time honored procedure for recovering gold and silver and basically, it's, it's been performed for 250-300 years. It's the accepted standard in the industry.

Ah, after we recovered this gold and silver for a couple of weeks, we began to recover something else. And the something else was recovering as if it's gold and silver but it wasn't gold and silver. Our beads of gold and silver were actually getting to the point that you could hit them with a hammer and they would shatter. Now there's no alloy of gold and silver that will become that brittle. Gold and silver are both very soft metals and they don't alloy in any proportion that would cause them to become hard or brittle. Yet this became very hard and brittle. When we sent it to the standard laboratories for analysis, all they could detect was gold and silver with traces, and just traces, of copper. Something was recovering with the gold and silver. We couldn't explain. And eventually it got so much of this in our recovery system that actually we were losing gold and silver when we recovered this other material. And so, you know, it wasn't supposed to be profitable, it's just supposed to be something that was interesting.

And so I said, "Shut the system down. You know, let's find out what the problem material really is". And chemically we were able to separate the "problem material" from the gold and silver and I had this sample of pure problem stuff, whatever it was. And you have to understand my background is cotton farming. I decided to go into agriculture but I hated chemistry, I hated physics, like most of you. And ah, I decided, well heck, you know if you just pay enough money to the right experts, you can hire enough PhD's, you'll be able to figure this problem out. So I went to Cornell University, where a man had written these papers on doing x-ray analysis and he took the sample of the problem material, which wouldn't dissolve in any acids or bases. It was cobalt blue in color. And he did an analysis on it and he told me it was iron silica and aluminum. I said it's not iron silica and aluminum. He said, "Well sorry that's what the analysis says it is". So, working within Cornell, we removed all of the iron, all the silica and all the aluminum from the sample. We still had over 98 percent of the sample. At this point he said, "Dave, it analyzes to be nothing". (audience laughter)

He said, "Mr. Hudson, if you'll give us a $350,000 grant, we'll put graduate students to working on it". Well I had paid him about $12,000 thus far. He told me he could analyze anything down to parts per billion and now he's telling me I had pure nothing. He didn't offer to refund any of my money and so I said, "No thank you, I think for $350,000 I can get more information than you can". That was about 1981 and basically I embarked on a research program of my own.

I said to myself, "you know, I am going to fund the thing myself and I am going to get the answers to it". [**End of David Hudson speaking**]

The Adventure Continues

So he did. David Hudson proceeded to spend years and several million more dollars researching the mysterious metallic substance that he had discovered. He even employed scientists and laboratories in England, Germany and Russia to assist him. Eventually it was discovered that his mystery element had hither-to-unknown physical properties. And eventually it was presented to David and his researchers that they had rediscovered an element that had been known by ancient civilizations. They also learned that these ancient civilizations had cherished this special element for its spiritual and rejuvenating powers. He first named his special element "the white powder of gold". Later he nicknamed the material "ormus" which was an abbreviation for "the orbitally rearranged monatomic elements of rhodium and iridium that exist in the presence of gold".

At this point in his adventure, David Hudson had spent eight million dollars of his own money on this project. Now he felt that he was ready to build an actual plant to manufacture his white powder of gold. But he needed to raise an additional five million dollars that would be required to build his ormus production plant. It was then that he spent three years touring the US, making personal presentations to interested groups. He raised his five million dollars by selling "shares" on his production project for $1,000 apiece. By 1996 he had his five million dollars, and construction started on a plant in Tempe, Arizona.

He sent out periodic progress reports to his investors. Each several months they received exciting news as his project headed toward completion. By the end of 1998 the plant was almost ready. Each investor had been promised a steady supply of the "white powder of gold". They waited expectantly. It was a time of jubilation and celebration. The years of waiting were about to pay off.

The week of the plant startup began. Then disaster struck. At 2:00am one morning, a force of 150 Federal agents swept into the plant, claiming that there was a gas leak of poisonous acid fumes that endangered the community. The plant was shut down. Then federal forces brought in a work force, dismantled the plant, cut all of the steel components into pieces, and hauled them off to an unknown destination. The metal factory building was torn down, cut up, and hauled away. Bulldozers tore apart the concrete foundation and hauled it off. All of this was done without any due process of law. What was left was the bare ground that had existed before David had bought the property. As one sarcastic observer remarked, "The government may have overreacted a bit."

David Hudson was simultaneously hit with massive lawsuits by the government. He suffered a massive heart attack. He sent out one last, sad, report to his investors telling them what had transpired. Then he dropped out of sight and has not reappeared publicly since.

I know all about this because I was one of his investors. During the years that the plant was under construction, I on several occasions had wondered if the government would allow this knowledge to be made public. Now I had my answer.

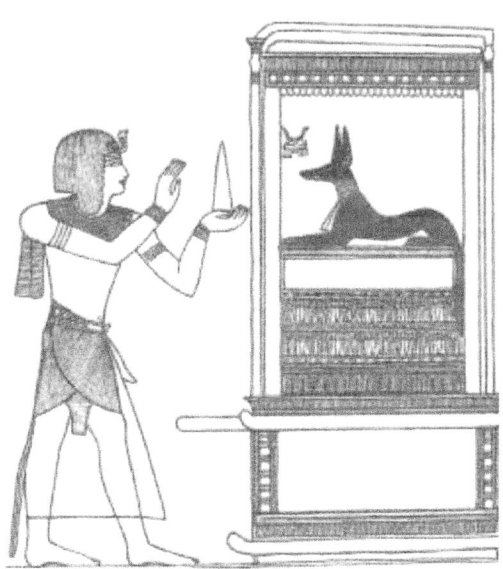

So this adventure, I thought to myself, is over. But I was wrong.

The Internet to the rescue!

Six months later something very interesting happened. Formulas for making the white powder of gold and ormus began to appear on several Internet websites. The instructions on these websites even told you how to make it in your kitchen.

Since then, numerous groups around the country have formed to study this material. There are "Ormus Workshops" held at numerous locations. Experimentations have abounded. New, simple methods of making ormus have evolved. Wonderful books such as "Lost Secrets of the Sacred Ark" by the distinguished European historian and researcher Laurence Gardner have hit the marketplace. The Internet abounds with articles, study-groups, DVDs and books on the subject.

So the knowledge of ormus has not been lost this time. But as I am sure that you realize, most of the people in the world are not ready for this knowledge. It seems that the ancients knew to keep knowledge of ormus restricted to the privilege ruling and priest classes. Likewise they restricted the use of it to a few highly select individuals (the priests and ruling families).

For instance, in ancient Egypt, only the Pharaohs and the High Priests could partake of their ormus. It was known to them as shewbread. The ormus was baked into conical loaves of bread that were used in special ceremonies. There are hieroglyphs and wall engravings in Egypt that show the conical loaves of shewbread being presented to the Pharaoh or one of the Gods.

Above is shown a mural picture of the Pharaoh presenting some shewbread to the God Anubis. This mural is at the Temple of Abydos.

Special Features of Ormus

As we progress into more detailed information about ormus, it is time to point out a few special things about ormus. As David Hudson continued to study his "orbitally rearranged molecules of rhodium and iridium that exist in the presence of gold", he and his researchers began to observe that this "ormus", whatever it was, had a consciousness. This was really weird. But, as researchers, they had the obligation to honor their observations.

Then they realized that their observations in this regard were totally consistent with ancient writing about this substance. It was the ancient Hebrew priests who would only let specially prepared priests into the presence of their stored ormus. And the ancient Hindu and Vedic texts also referred to the fact that only those who were properly spiritually prepared could prepare the elixir.

And it was the alchemists of the middle ages who always insisted that only the "pure of heart" and those with "purity of intent" who could make the philosopher's stone.

Suddenly all of this began to make sense. Because this mysterious element, whatever it was, had consciousness, it could sense the consciousness of the people about it. And apparently this mysterious substance, that we arbitrarily now refer to as "ormus", chooses to be around people of a higher quality of consciousness. This is very important when it comes to preparing ormus products. Simply put, the higher the quality of consciousness of the preparer, the greater the quantity, and the higher quality of the ormus that is produced.

So when you begin to take ormus, you want to be sure that a person who has a positive mind and is spiritually balanced has produced the ormus. It is also very important that the preparer "declare, or set, his intent to the ormus before he attempts to precipitate it into his product. In this regard, a properly balanced preparer will always say a prayer before beginning his preparation process, asking all of the angelic and nature forces to assist him in his endeavor.

Researchers also eventually discovered that there is ormus in everything. Some things have more ormus than others. For instance, grapes have an extraordinarily large amount of ormus in them. So does the brains of newborn babies. Water has ormus in it, especially water that carries minute amounts of gold and silver in it. Sea Water, heavily laden with minerals including gold and silver, is a treasure trove for the ormus producer.

Other features of ormus that are important to understand are that ormus is sensitive to bright light, electrical fields and magnetic fields. So I always try to keep my stored ormus away from bright lights. Likewise I do not store it near electrical appliances or electrical wires. The feature of ormus that it does not like magnetic fields is especially important to understand, because we utilize this feature to "capture" ormus out of water with our ormus magnetic water trap.

Here is how it works: Since ormus does not like magnetic fields, we run a lot of water past a magnet. The water passes the magnetic field without incident, but the ormus that is present in the water does not want to go past the magnet. So it stays behind. In other words, the ormus accumulates in the water that is "upstream" of the magnet. Clever people have invented gizmos that will capture this accumulated ormus. They are known as "ormus accumulators" or "ormus water traps". We will discuss this much more as we continue.

The Ormus Experience

When you are ready to try ormus, there are a number of ways that you can proceed. I shall discuss each of these ways.

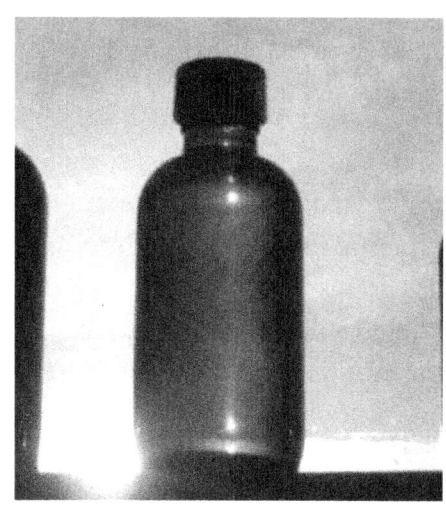

1. Buy Ormus from a supplier on the Internet.
2. Make your own Ormus water with a magnetic water trap.
3. Make your own Ormus with sacred geometry cylinders.
4. Make your own Ormus using the Wet Method.

Buying Ormus from a supplier on the Internet

Probably the best way for you to begin your adventure with ormus is for you to buy some ormus. The Internet is the way to do this.

Simply go to your favorite search engine and search the keywords "ormus", "ormes (another word for ormus), "white powder of gold", or "David Hudson". There are plenty of websites out there that deal with ormus. Probably the premium website is http://subtleenergies.com . This is the website of Barry Carter.

Barry Carter is a wonderful and pure man. He picked up the mantle after David Hudson went underground, and it is primarily due to Barry's unselfish work that the word of ormus has spread so far and wide. He has spent years touring the country, conducting workshops and talks about ormus. He presents internet forums about ormus. His website has grown to where it is the definitive source of information about ormus. Barry has never made a lot of money doing this. He just seems to do it because someone has to do it. Thank God for Barry Carter.

On his website Barry will recommend reliable sources of ormus. All of them are good and reliable. But my favorite is Don Nance. His website is http://oceanalchemy.com . I recommend that a beginner start with his "Great Salt Lake Manna". An 8 oz. bottle costs $50. This is a pretty much standard price. I started with this product. It is great for the beginner. Two weeks on this ormus and your world will begin to change right in front of your eyes. I recommend that you begin by taking ½ teaspoon of ormus twice daily, and gradually work up to a larger dose.

Why do I recommend Don Nance? Because I know him personally, and I know that he has a pure heart and puts very pure intent into his products as he makes them. I also recommend him because he is one of the ormus pioneers who has unselfishly taught and guided many others such as myself as we struggled to learn the amazing truths about ormus.

After you have begun taking ormus that you have purchased from a supplier on the Internet, you may then find that you are ready to tackle the challenge of making ormus yourself. My suggestion, based on my own experiences, is that you next begin to make your own ormus using an ormus water trap.

The Ormus Water Trap

After one of our ingenious ormus pioneers figured out that you could use the fact that ormus avoided magnetic fields to "separate" out ormus from regular tap water, a variety of types of ormus water traps began to appear in the Internet. Some gracious inventors even present detailed instructions (with pictures) on how to make your own water trap. I did this. It is a lot of work, and the parts cost a lot of money. It is much simpler to just buy one. Shown on this page is a picture of one of the water traps that is for sale in the Internet. It costs about $200. But it will last for a lifetime. Not a bad investment.

How do you use it? Simple. You hook it up to a hose connection at your house, put a gallon jug on the other end, and turn it on. Now wait about 24 hours. During those 24 hours, about

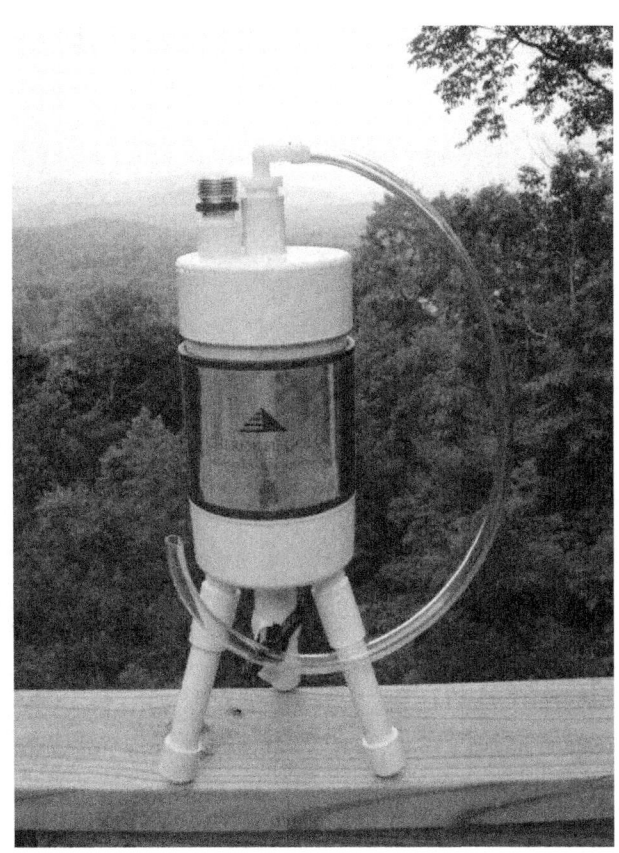

4,000 gallons of water will have run through the water trap, leaving behind the ormus that was present in the 4,000 gallons. So now you have a gallon of water that collected the ormus that was present on 4,000 gallons of water. This is your accumulated ormus water.

Store this water safely. Shown on this page is a glass water bottle wrapped in two layers of aluminum foil, and then given a protective wrapping of duct tape [hey, I had to get duct tape in here somewhere! (smile)]. This is where I store my ormus water, protecting it from light, electrical and magnetic waves. I keep it in the pantry. I drink half a glass, twice daily.

My ormus water trap served me nicely for seven years. But I eventually got frustrated with wasting 4,000 gallons of water each time I made ormus. I have a well at my home, so this wasn't too bad. And my septic system meant that the water went right back into the local aquifer. So in a sense my water wasn't really wasted. But for my friends who were using city water, and paid for their metered water, the ormus water trap used a lot of water.

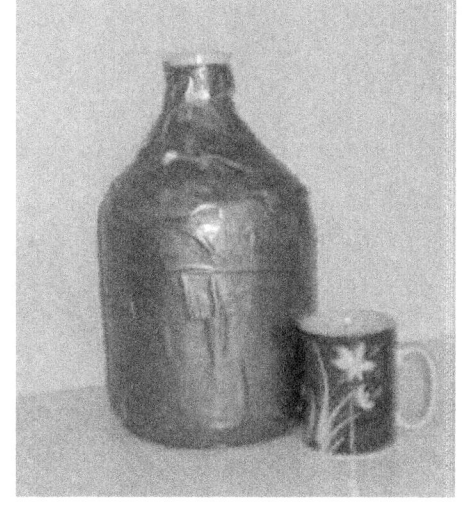

So when people such as Barry carter and Don Nance and Chris Emmons (another pioneer) began to show me other ways of making ormus, I continued on with my own ormus education.

Shape Has Power: Using Sacred Geometry to make Ormus Water

This method of making ormus water is different from anything we have discussed. It uses the principles of sacred geometry to gather ormus from the universe. Please remember that we have discussed that the elements of matter that comprise what we know as ormus has a consciousness, and also seems to have an aversion to bright light, electrical fields and magnetic fields.

We have used their aversion to magnetic fields to utilize a magnetic water trap to separate out the ormus that is found in ordinary drinking water. Thus we have made magnetic trap water. What we are just now realizing is that the ormus particles also have a consciousness. This explains why the ancient alchemists had to have purity of intent when they did their work, why the ancient Hindu gurus had to pray over their work, and why the European alchemists insisted on purity of intent in their work.

A Short Explanation of the Powers of Sacred geometry

Now we will use the consciousness of the ormus matter to capture it in water. In this, we will use the principles of ancient Egyptian sacred geometry.

What is sacred geometry?

Wikipedia Defines Sacred Geometry: Wikipedia, the Internet dictionary, defines sacred geometry as follows: Sacred geometry is geometry used in the design of sacred architecture and sacred art. The basic belief is that geometry and mathematical ratios, harmonics and proportion are also found in music, light, and cosmology. This value system is seen as widespread even in prehistory, a cultural universal of the human condition. It is considered foundational to building sacred structures such as temples, mosques, megaliths, monuments and churches; sacred spaces such as altars, temenoi and tabernacles; meeting places such as sacred groves, village greens and holy wells, religious art, iconography and using "divine" 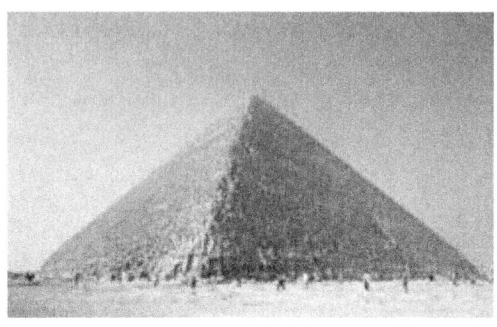 proportions. We, the western societies, experienced this knowledge of Sacred geometry briefly. For when the Templars returned from the crusades in the 13th and 14th centuries they brought this knowledge with them. They had studied at the ancient Egyptian Mystery Schools, and they had access to this knowledge. The most famous cathedrals of Europe were built during this period. Even today we cannot duplicate the mystical and tranquilizing effects experienced by people who stand in the presence of their awesome power.

Basically, as I explain it, the universe is constructed using certain principles of harmonics and rules of proportion. If you are aware of this, it is possible to use these principles to capture beneficial forces from the universe. If you have designed a building that follows these harmonic proportions, the building will have beneficial energies that other buildings do not. As has been observed in the ancient cathedrals of Europe that were built by the Templars, people who stand in these structures "feel better" and have a great sense of peace and harmony.

After the Crusades, the Templars built cathedrals all over Europe using sacred geometry. These cathedrals are now famous. It is actually the harmony and perfect proportions of these edifices, not their fancy detail, that cause them to be still so widely visited by thousands of tourists each year. In later centuries, other, more elaborate cathedrals and churches were built, but they lack the power of the edifices built according to the rules of harmony and proportion as taught by the

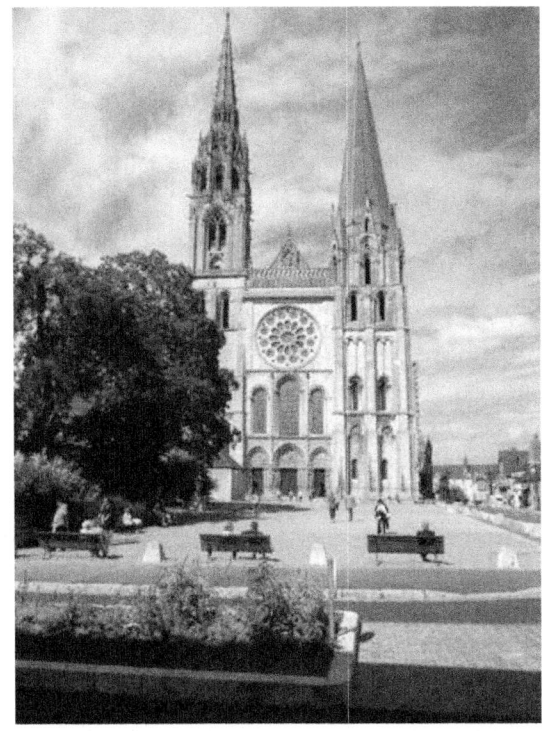

Egyptians. For when the Templars were destroyed in 1307, their knowledge
was mostly lost to the world.

  Briefly, in a nutshell, what I learned is that there are sacred dimensions that resonate with the creative forces of the universe. The ancient Egyptians knew of this knowledge. They built their temples and municipal buildings according to these rules, using a knowledge of sacred geometry that many believe was brought to them from Atlantis. This sacred geometry was known to ancient civilizations in India, Central and South America, and elsewhere. The Taj Mahal is every bit as much an example of this ancient wisdom as is the Great Pyramid. What these ancient civilizations knew is that buildings built using the universal laws of sacred design would enhance the physical being of the people who occupied these buildings. Somehow special energies that exist in the universe are drawn to or amplified in these structures so that the overall health, sense of well-being and spiritual balance of those people who inhabit the structures are enhanced.

To the Egyptians, the square and the circle were their two most powerful shapes. Shown on this page is a house in India that is built on this principle. The central patio and the house dimensions are perfect squares.

A three-dimensional extension of the circle is the cylinder. A cylinder, by the very nature of its perfect harmony, attracts beneficial energies from the universe. For a reason that we do not understand, it also attracts ormus elements. They apparently like to "hang out" in a cylinder. We do not know why, we just know that they do.

So we stumbled onto a really great way to make ormus water. It works. We don't know why. It just works.

This is a great way to make ormus water because:

1. There is almost no cost.
2. It does not waste any water, as does the magnetic water trap method.
3. It is simple and inexpensive to build the cylinders that you need for this method.
4. It uses discarded wine bottles and cardboard cylinders, PVC pipe, or coffee cans for the cylinders. All are readily available.

Proof that it works.

When I began to use this method, I was skeptical. It was too easy. How could something so easy to build and use work? I was drinking the water. It seemed to be working on me. But measuring such things is subjective. I wanted some proof that was more independent.

So I did an experiment. It was winter. I took two clay flower pots, added potting soil and some cucumber seeds. I set them up in front of a window in my house. A picture of the two pots is shown. Then I watered the pot on the left with water that had spent three days in my three concentric cylinders. I watered the pot on the right with untreated water. The results, shown after ten days, are dramatic.

I strongly recommend that you do a similar experiment yourself. It is easy to do, and is cheap. And it will do wonders to remind you that what you are doing works!

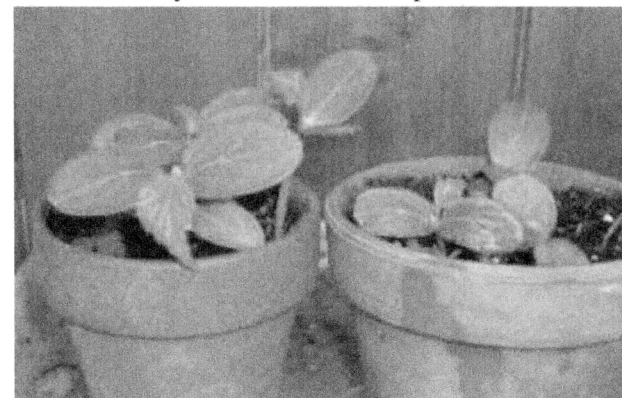

How My Three Cylinder Method Works:

I like to build my cylinders using cardboard mailing tubes for the cylinders. But I have also used PVC pipe, tin cans, what-have you. What is important is the shape, and it doesn't seem to matter what the cylinders are made of. I first used just one cylinder. It took a week for the water to be fully energized with ormus. Then I found that if I used three cylinders, each one inside the other, that the treatment time was cut to three days. So that is the method that I use now. Shown above is one of my three-cylinder systems. I use an empty 1.5 liter wine bottle, filled with water. I store it in the cylinders for three days. I have eight of these 3-cylinder systems in use. They fill one shelf in the kitchen pantry. I try to drink at least one-half of a bottle of this treated water daily.

I start out each morning using this water to make my coffee. Boiling doesn't seem to bother the ormus. Then, during the day, I drink water from the bottle as I get thirsty. As time progresses, you will be able to drink more and more of the water. The more that you drink, of course, the faster you will get results.

I ordered my mailing tubes off of the Internet. I used Yahoo Mills as my supplier. I ordered 5 inch diameter, six inch diameter, and eight inch diameter mailing tubes. I cut them to a length of 12 inches. The cost of enough tubing to make my eight 3-cylinder systems was about $200. This is not cheap. But then again, these systems should last me for the rest of my life. Some of my friends have used discarded carpet roll cores to make their cylinders.

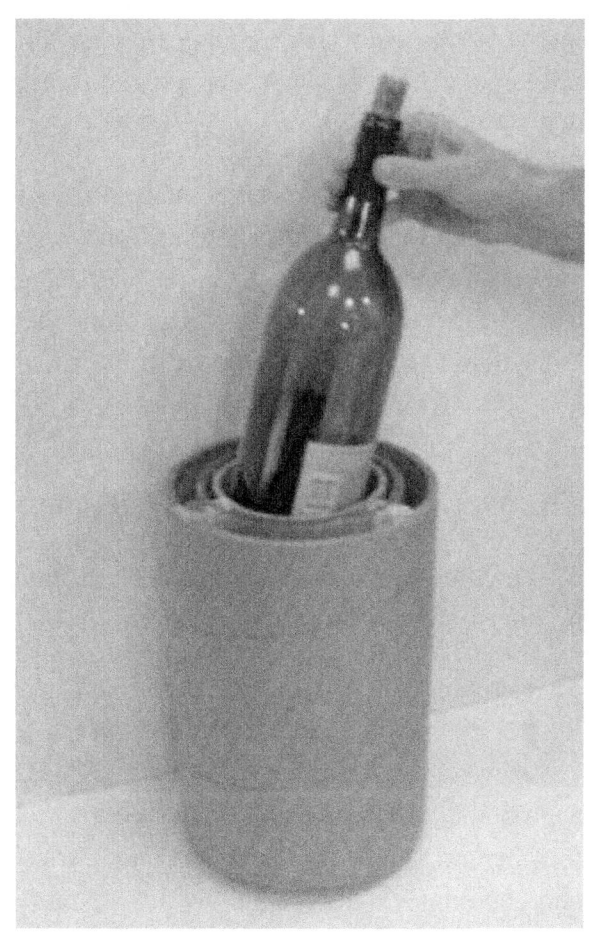

I also cut some old wine bottle corks into short pieces that I glued (using construction adhesive) between the cylinders to hold then all in place. You can see this in the above picture.

Well, this form of ormus that is made in concentric cylinders is very helpful. It will extend longevity and give you many health benefits. It helped me greatly. But I gradually, after a number of years of only drinking this ormus water, realized that I also needed to take another stronger form of ormus in order to reach the goals of longevity and spiritual balance that I sought.

Thus it was that I also began to make a stronger ormus product that I consumed in conjunction with my sacred cylinder water. This stronger ormus is made using what is called "the wet method". It extracts ormus from sea water. We will discuss this method now.

The Wet Method of making Ormus

This method will make for you the same ormus that you previously bought from Don Nance.

This simple method can be done in your kitchen. It is called the wet method because it is made from sea water (or Great Lakes water), or a mixture of water and fresh sea salt. There are a number of recipes on the Internet that tell how to use this method to make an ormus product. I tried many of them, and I could never get them to work. Therefore for year after year I stuck with using ormus water made from my ormus magnetic trap.

Then I attended an ormus conference in 2009. One of the presenters was a wonderful man by the name of Don Nance. His talk to us was good, but what really blew me away was the generosity and lovingness with which he readily shared all of his knowledge with us. As I have previously mentioned, Don makes an ormus product that he sells on the Internet. Therefore one could assume that he would be reluctant to share his secrets with the world. Not so. He freely gave us wonderful and detailed instructions, as he personally demonstrated to us his wet method process. So now that is the process that I personally use. And that is the process that I am going to show you now.

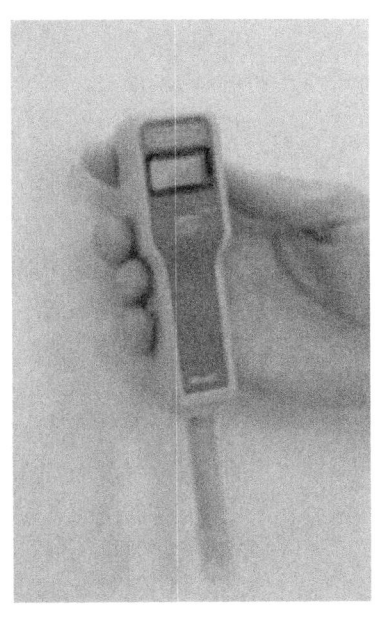

You will need the following:

1. A large glass mixing bowl, at least 5 qt. capacity.
2. A hand-held ph meter. The one shown here costs about $40.00 and I bought it off the Internet. Be sure to get one that reads from the 7.0 to 12.0 ph range.
3. Two wooden clothespins, glued together as shown, to hold the ph meter in the bowl. This frees up both of your hands for the mixing operation.
4. A pint (16 oz.) of concentrated and purified sea water or Great Lakes salt water. The bottle shown cost less than $10.00 and was found on the Internet. If you choose to try regular salt water, it will have to be carefully boiled and filtered to remove all impurities, and you will use 32 oz. of regular sea water.

5. A non-metallic stirrer. A regular kitchen plastic spoon works. I use a cheap wooden paint stirrer that is 12 inches long.

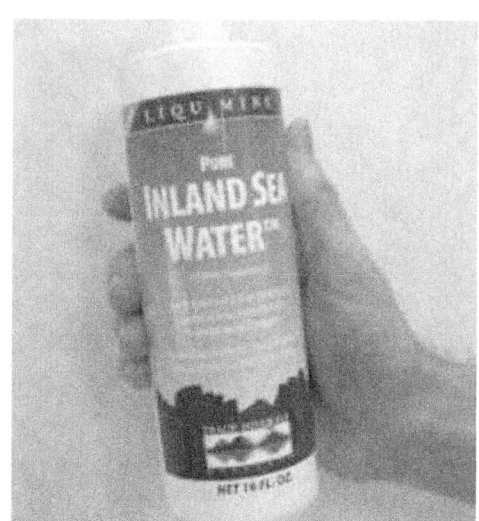

6. A glass measuring cup, at least one-cup capacity.
7. Pure lye (sodium hydroxide). I bought mine from a science supply company on the internet. The government has started making the Red Devil Lye Company put ingredients in their lye so it is no longer safe to use Red Devil Lye. Some people buy their lye from plumbing supply stores.
8. Two gallons of pure distilled water. I buy mine at the grocery store and pay about $1.00 per gallon. It is important to use pure distilled water because not only is it clean, it has no minerals in it that might interfere with the chemical reactions.
9. A small bottle of white distilled vinegar. This will be used in an emergency, should you accidently raise the ph of your mixture past 10.78. You will immediately add a small amount of the vinegar (an acid) to reduce the ph back down below 10.78.

10. About 4 ft. of clear 3/8 inch plastic tubing.

The Process

1. Add the 16 oz. bottle of sea mineral water to the bowl.
2. The distilled water should be a room temperature. Now add the distilled water to the bowl. Fill the mixing bowl to within 1.5 inches of the top with distilled water.
3. Put two teaspoons of powdered lye into the small glass measuring cup. Now add 16 teaspoons (the ratio is 8 times as much water as there is lye) of water to the cup, and gently shake to mix. Heat should be given off as the water and lye mix. Note: Never add lye to water, it may explode and burn your eyes or skin. Water and lye can be dangerous. It will burn your eyes, skin

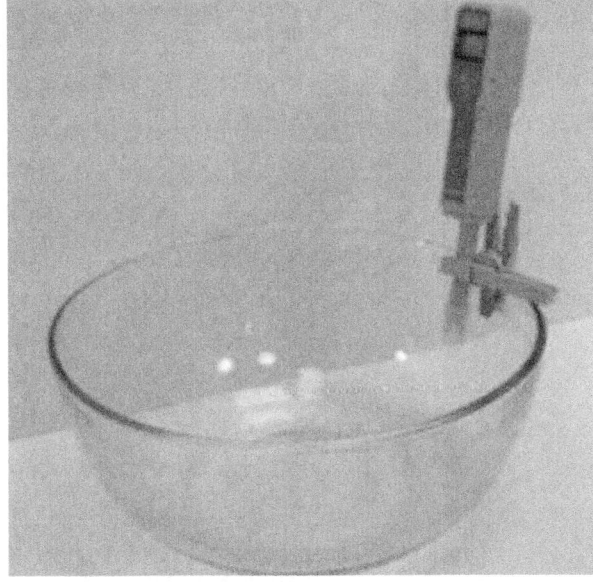

and clothing if you are not careful.

4. Turn the calibrated ph meter on and mount it in the wooden clothespin holder on the side of the bowl.

5. Check the ph of the water in the large mixing bowl. It should be somewhere between 7.5 and 9.0.

6. Now the most important and critical part. You must be very patient and methodical. If you try to rush this, you may ruin your batch. **Do this part very slowly.** Begin to stir the mixture of water with the mixing spoon. Now slowly pour a very small trickle of lye water from the measuring cup into the bowl as you continue stirring. From now on, you must continuously stir the water until the target ph of 10.7 is reached. Watch the ph meter carefully. As you very slowly add the lye water, the ph of the mixture should slowly rise. The emphasis is to pour **slowly!** Keep stirring the mixture at all times to insure that the ph meter is getting a correct reading of the exact ph of the mixture. As you do this, you may observe the phenomenon that there are "level spots" in the ph reading. This means that you will get to a spot where, as you continue to add lye water, the ph does not go up. Be very carefully here. You have hit a level spot. The tendency here is to get impatient and add too much lye water. This will be a mistake, because once the level spot has been passed, the ph may just jump dramatically.

7. Your objective is to get the mixture raised to a ph of exactly 10.78. Many ph meters will read to only 10.7. This is good enough! Actually, when you get the mixture to a point where the ph meter fluctuates

between 10.6 and 10.7 you are finished. This is good enough. You can stop now. What happens now is that the monatomic elements of gold, silver, rhodium, iridium and platinum settle out of the sea water when the ph gets to around 10.6 to 10.7

8. If you accidently get the ph of your mixture to 10.8 or above, quickly add a small amount of white vinegar to bring the ph down again below 10.7, and start over.

9. Once you have your mixture at a steady ph of 10.6 to 10.7 you are finished. You will notice that a white material has begun to settle out of the water. This white material is the monatomic form of gold and other precious metals that is precipitated from the precious metals that naturally exist in the sea water.

10. At this point you must wait from 4 to 6 hours for the white material to finish precipitating. I usually wait overnight for this to happen. I place a large inverted platter over the mixing bowl to protect the ingredients, and then cover everything with a towel to keep light out.

11. The next morning you will notice that the white precipitate is now concentrated in the bottom 1/3 of the bowl. This wet white precipitate is what you want to harvest. So, using the 4 ft. piece of 3/8 inch plastic tubing, carefully siphon as much of the clear water out of the bowl as is possible without disturbing the white precipitate on the bottom. My procedure is to place one end of the clear plastic tubing in the same wooden clothespin holder that I used to hold the ph meter. Then I adjust the end of the tubing so that it rests about 3/16 in. above the white precipitate. Then I

place the other end of the tubing into a white plastic 5 gallon bucket that is on the floor. Suck on that end until the flow of water starts, then place that end into the bucket as the clear water drains out of the mixing bowl.

12. You will be left with the layer of white precipitate in water plus about 3/16 inch of clear water above it. This is the final product. Pour it into a pitcher and then store in glass bottles. I wrap my bottles in aluminum foil to protect the precipitate as much as possible from magnetic and electrical fields.

This is it. Now you have made a 4 to 6 week supply of ormus precipitate that is powerful and effective. Begin by taking ½ teaspoon twice daily and gradually build up to two tablespoons twice daily. The cost for this 4 to 6 week supply will be about $10.00. Not bad!

Further notes:

1. Many people choose to take their bowl that has the wet precipitate in it and add more distilled water to refill the bowl. They stir the mixture again. Then they repeat the settling process, again draining off the excess water. They may do this 3 or 4 times. This is called "washing" the precipitate. It removes most of the salty taste from the precipitate.

2. I prefer to not "wash" the precipitate. I have several reasons for this. First of all, I like the salty taste. And the natural sea salt is healthy for you, giving you beneficial minerals and trace elements from the sea water. But there is a more important reason. The salt

in the mix protects the ormus particles from damage by light, electrical and magnetic fields. For some reason, the ormus likes to "hide out" in the salt matrix. So by leaving the salt in the mix, you have a better and stronger ormus product, with an improved shelf life.

Conclusion and Summary

Well, this has been a wild ride, hasn't it? Your belief systems have really taken a beating. It is really difficult for most people to accept what you have just read. I understand this myself, because I too had to go through this torturous tunnel when I first began this journey.

Congratulations to you for being courageous and brave. Yes, you are courageous and brave if you have made it to this point in the booklet!

This information could, of necessity, only be a brief overview of this very complex subject. Many questions may flood your head after you have read this material. I hope that you will use the wonderful abilities of the Internet and also the books listed in the Bibliography as starting points to do a more complete research of this fascinating discovery of ormus.

As I delved deeply into this subject, I gradually came to the realization that most people cannot handle this information because they are not, at this time in mankind's development, ready for this information.

Just as in ancient times, a small number of people are allowed access to this life altering information. But there is an important difference this time. In ancient times it was the high priest and the nobility who were entitled to partake of the white powder of gold. Now, in today's world, it is the brave adventurer, the seeker of truth, the most intelligent of people, who are allowed to access this knowledge. I like this. It certainly seems more fair!

So my best wishes to you as you begin your own exciting journey. I am enclosing in the Addendum several photos and several testimonials that may provide some additional value to you.

And yes, one final (and very wild) thought that I wish to share with you (I just can't help myself!). As I worked with this strange stuff called ormus, and as I accepted that it had a consciousness, I gradually began to be aware that it is friendly. Then, finally, the awesome truth hit me. I believe that ormus is a "love component" of the universe. I now believe that ormus is something that God created that is part of his awesome love that he has for us. I realized that ormus loves us, and wants to help us. That is why when you pray over your ormus-making process, you get more ormus than otherwise. That is why if you ask it to help you, your results will be better. That is why the ancients knew that ormus should only be made by those of a pure heart. Love is attracted to love. So let's go for the love!

Bibliography

Laurence Gardner, *Lost Secrets of the sacred Ark*, ISBN 0-767-7598-2

Robert E. Cox, *the Elixir of Immortality*, ISBN 978-159477303-7

Chris Emmons, *Ormus Modern Day Alchemy*, ISBN 978-0-9815840-1-0

Henry Kroll, *The Philosopher Stone; Immortality Discovered* ISBN 1-932672-24-9

R.A. Schwaller de Lubicz, *Sacred Science*, ISBN 0-89281-222-2

A Treatise: How Ormus repairs DNA and how it works

This information in this section is extracted from the book *The Philosopher Stone* by Henry Kroll.

In order for body cells to replicate they have to split the genes of the old cell to produce a new cell, the old cell sharing the genes with the new cell. The process of "unzipping" the gene codes completely, without damaging the gene codes, requires that certain minerals be present. These minerals are the monatomic mineral state of gold and platinum.

This critical process is made more difficult in these modern times because of our mineral-deficient diets. The soils that most of our vegetables and fruits are grown on have long-ago become deficient in most of the 84 minerals and trace elements that we need for perfect health. Linus Pauling, two-time Nobel Prize winner, stated, "You can trace every sickness, every disease and every ailment to a mineral deficiency".

Each time a cell replicates, it loses a few of the gene chains called tellimires. When enough of the tellimires are gone, the cell dies. Thus it is the loss of these tellimires in the body cells that causes aging. If a cell has enough of the right superconducting minerals during cell replication it doesn't lose any tellimires. Therefore it can replicate indefinitely.

If a person's body is saturated with monatomic-state elements of gold and platinum, it is possible for a person to live for hundreds of years free of disease and without the problems of aging. [Perhaps this helps to explain the Old Testament people who were reported to live for many hundreds of years.]

In addition, the monatomic-state silver minerals in Ormus also play an important part in your health. The monatomic silver elements are tied to the very process of life itself. Monatomic silver kills disease organisms, promotes major growth of bone, and accelerates the healing of body tissue. It also speeds up the cell replication process.

Concerning the type of people who are able to accept ormus into their lives, Mr. Kroll states, "Some people are drawn into this knowledge from a very deep part of their soul". Enough said. If you are reading this, this probably means you.

Moses had several methods of making manna. When they were travelling in the desert, he and his brother Aaron took desert soil that was high in alkalinity and boiled it in alkaline water for several days. As the water boiled away, they added more alkaline water that they got from certain desert springs, making the brew even more alkaline. They then cooled the high-alkaline mixture and added vinegar to drop the ph. As the ph dropped, a milky substance formed. This was the monatomic states of the precious metals previously mentioned. The clear liquid was poured off, and the milky substance that was left over was their manna. This milky liquid was baked into whatever grains they had with them, and the resulting loaves were their "shewbread", their life-sustaining food that got them through the desert wilderness.

Anyone who has made Ormus using the Wet Method will be impressed with the similarities between these two methods.

Section B: Viktor Shauberger and his Energized Water:

The best way for us to proceed here is for you to read the book "Living Energies" by Callum Coats (available on amazon.com). The fascinating and adventurous life of Viktor Shauberger is well worth reading. And you should know about his discoveries. When you pull the plug on your bathtub, and the water makes a spiraling motion as it exits through the drain, the water is forming this spin in a natural motion to energize itself. It is the same pattern that we see in tornadoes. Keep this simple example in mind, for it explains much about Shauberger's discoveries.

Many do, as I have, set up a device to spin the water as it enters our homes through the water pipes. I suggest that you may well choose to also do this. The Internet will show devices that you can put on your water pipes to accomplish this.

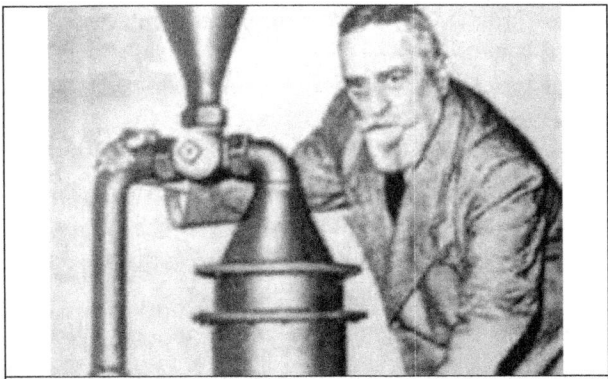

Viktor Shauberger shows off one of his energy inventions.

However there is a severe limitation to this. The water does not store this energy. It is soon lost. Therefore it is not possible to "bottle" this energy for later use. Thus I am not going to spend much time on it.

However it is important to understand the principles taught by Viktor Shauberger.

Here is a special treat. This utube video shows devices using Shauberger technology and Emoto knowledge to create special water:
http://www.youtube.com/watch?v=YVL6tfGhr8M

Section C: The development of Cancell water:

Note: This is a reprint of an article that appeared in Nexus Magazine January 1994:

Curing AIDS and Cancer
Interview with Ed Sopcak

CanCell is a carrier of vibrational frequencies which, despite being unapproved by the FDA, has cured AIDS, cancer, and other diseases.

Nexus Magazine, December-January 1994	Taken from vol 1, no 31 of Sovereign Scribe Magazine, PO Box 350, McKenna, WA 98558, USA. Phone 206 458 2699

ES: Ed Sopcak (pronounced 'Soap-check').

SS: *Sovereign Scribe.*

SS: How did you get first get involved in his type of work?

ES: I was working with free energy devices which is all about vibrational frequencies. During this time I had a friend named Don over at the University of Michigan who was at Saint Joseph's, who was a terminal cancer patient. They gave him six weeks to live. He got a hold of a product from Jim Sheridan called Entelev. He took that while at St Joseph's and ended up without any cancer in six weeks. That gets one's attention.

Now Jim Sheridan had started on the research project Entelev back in 1936. By 1947 he felt that he had a workable model that would cure about 38% of all cancer. He kept working. The more successful he got, the more unhappy the FDA got with him. So by the time 1984 came around he had had it; he quit and decided nobody wanted it and he just wasn't going to do it anymore. So this friend of mine asked me if I would make it for him. I said sure, get me the formulation and I would make it. So he did. Now Jim was looking at it from a chemical standpoint, having himself a degree in physical chemistry. I started looking at it from a standpoint of basic vibrational physics. So I made a few minor changes in the formulation based on vibrational physics. I made some and gave it to my friend. Then others heard about it who were terminal cancer patients and we gave it to them. This continued to grow. I've been at it for 10 years now.

All cancer is an anaerobic cell that has mutated. Cancer is a single disease. With the application of Entelev, Jim took an anaerobic cell and pushed it back through primitive, which meant it went back to the amino acids the body used to create the protein in the first place.

Now everybody recognises that a cancer cell is an anaerobic cell. This is not news to anybody. The general attempt by people in cancer therapy is to take that weakened anaerobic cell and make it stronger with vitamins or whatever, and try to push it back to being an aerobic cell. You can't do that. Jim recognised this and his view was, rather than to make the cell healthy, he decided to just get rid of it. So he worked with the blockages within the enzyme system or the respiratory system and then he pushed the cell back through primitive and ended up with the amino acids that the body uses to create itself, and therefore the cancer no longer existed.

SS: Is this related to the hydrogen peroxide approach of creating an oxygen-rich environment whereby anaerobic cells can't function?

ES: Technically, but the first thing you must understand about hydrogen peroxide or these others is that nothing works chemically. Everything on the face of the Earth is electromagnetic vibrational frequency. Therefore, when you get into peroxide there's the assumption that since the formulation is H_2O_2, that it will always break to H_2O + oxygen and that is not true. It can also break into 2 OH radicals and very often does. But if it works for you, take it. If it doesn't, don't.

SS: So the vibrational changes brought about by CanCell, are these vibrations higher or lower?

ES: It starts out with a very high vibration and it degenerates over a 12-hour period. In doing that, as it comes down, it matches or gets into an interference pattern with viruses like the AIDS virus. It causes the virus to disassociate like the Memorex commercial with the glass when someone hits the note and the glass shatters. Well that's what happens with the virus.

SS: How does this relate with Rife's work?

ES: This is probably 50 to 75 years past the Rife technologies. We are now in a position on this planet where if anything plugs into a wall or uses a magnet to create the frequencies of the energy force, I would be suspect of it because the densities are too great We're working with high and extremely subtle frequencies. These frequencies cannot be measured with the technology we have today.

SS: So did you continue and advance the work of Jim Sheridan?

ES: I made CanCell for 6 months before I ever met Jim. We've been friends ever since meeting and I have a great deal of respect for him. We actually established a frequency that was a little above the frequency of oxygen. Not all oxygen has the same frequency. So what I believe that Jim was doing was starting out with a 6-ring organic compound and then he was manipulating the organic rings from 6 to 5 to 3 and various ratios. As you do this, every time you go from a 6- to a 5-ring compound, you increase the vibrational frequency. So he was really using chemicals to create a vibrational frequency in the water. So if you were able to take the dark material that Jim was making in the Entelev or early CanCell and you could filter out all of the dark materials, the material would still work. The chemistry had nothing to do with the function of the material. The only thing it had to do with was to create the frequency change.

So when we got to the point where the frequencies that I needed were higher than the frequencies I could get by the manipulation of chemicals, then we went to the new, improved CanCell several years ago. The new material analyses as pure water. The FDA told one of the doctors, so I hear, that they had run a clinical trial on CanCell. They found that it did everything I said it did. They figured there had to be something in the solution so they admitted that they tried using every known filter and couldn't filter anything out of it.   Then they made a conscious decision that they would use the power of the US Government in order to prevent the American citizens from knowing anything as simple as pure water that had been programmed could cure many different illnesses. This is the condition it is in today.

SS: So how do you alter the frequency of the water?

ES: Well the frequency of water gets changed every time it rains or anytime you put it up against anything. In other words, water is a programmable crystal. If anyone doubts that, ask yourself where do snowflakes come from? A change in a physical state doesn't change the crystalline structure.

So the first thing you have to do, since water has been on this planet for 10.5 million years, you have to get the memory or the history of what the water molecule remembers out of there. You must deprogramme the crystal and get it as close to a blank as you can. Then you can reprogramme it with the frequencies that you want. You erase the memory with a distillation process. After the water is distilled and clean and the memory is taken out of it, then I just simply place another memory into it.

SS: The water will retain this new memory?

ES: Yes. It depends on what you do. You can get both stable and unstable memories in it. That's one of the catches. The other catch is to get something that will work as CanCell does as a vibrational catalyst, so that if you simply get it in the aura of the body it will function. You do not have to take it internally or let it wet the skin. All you have to do is put it on a cotton pad and close to pulse points on the body. If you do that you will pick up the frequency from the CanCell. It will align die frequency of the aura. This affects the frequency of the cell structure. Once you have a balance in the cell structure then the body will cure itself. Cancell doesn't cure anything. All CanCell does is to allow the body to put itself into harmonic and vibrational balance.

SS: So what exactly is the cause of cancer?

ES: That's easy. As I said it is a mutation of an anaerobic cell. So where does that anaerobic cell come from? There are basically two sources of them. One is if you eat any fat or oil that carries a lot of free radicals. The free radicals affect the nucleic acids and will reproduce themselves in a damaged state. Free radicals are in any partially hydrogenated things such as margarine, disco or all the oils on the shelves. Also most baked goods have partially hydrogenated oil in them. This is the basic cause of an anaerobic cell

Another thing is if you eat protein. Protein digestion is a two-stage process in the body. At the end of the first stage of digestion you will have a DNA chemical or frequency that will damage the nucleic acid, and unless you have an adequate supply of vitamin B6 within the system you don't complete the digestion of protein. Therefore you will damage those nucleic acids and you will have the production of cells in a damaged state. When they are damaged enough, when they are sitting in a voltage range of between a negative .17 volts and a negative .21 volts, and when you have in the system a bacteria that's classified as a progenitor crypto-cyden, then that will facilitate the change of an aerobic cell to an anaerobic cell. Once you have anaerobic cells in the body those cells will create energy. You do come up with ATP but it's in a different form or ratio. When the body recognizes that you're coming in with a different ratio, why then the function of the body is to circle the wagon to protect itself.

This is where all of the degenerative diseases occur, such as arthritis, lupus, diabetes, M.S., Alzheimer's, Parkinson's, etc. They will stay there and create all kinds of mischief. Now if, at the same time, some place along the line the body has a chronic demand for energy that is greater than the cell structure is programmed to deliver, the body answers that demand for energy by mutating the anaerobic cells. Since the mutation of an anaerobic cell is cancer, that's the cause. Usually the chronic demand for energy here is stress. Over the past 10 years I've spoken to over 40,000 people with cancer. Almost universally, at least 90% of the time you can say to a person diagnosed with cancer, "Within 6 months to 3 years ago, you went through a stressful situation. What was it?" They always then say, "Well how did you know that?" It is almost chiselled in stone that that is the case.

SS: This leads us to the approach taken by people like Dr. Bernie Seigal who say that cancer is related to one's attitude.

ES: He is correct. Now when I used to answer the phone about 4 hours a day, volunteers have since taken over this for me, but I could tell simply by talking to the person with a 95% degree of accuracy whether CanCell could be used successfully for them or not. A person who takes CanCell and has cancer and is still staytag in a stressful situation, CanCell won't affect them at all. A person who is uptight and refuses to relinquish their stress, there's a problem there.

SS: Getting into a preventative approach, do free radical scavengers like vitamin E and SOD work?

ES: They sure do. Any of the antioxidants such as the B vitamins. Vitamin C, the water soluble one, and vitamin E, the oil soluble one, do work. The mineral is selenium. I don't personally take supplements of any type. I don't believe God put me here to be popping pills so I don't take things like that. But in general if you got your diet back to as much raw fruits and vegetables and nuts and minimally cooked foods, and if you did that and stayed away from animal products, I think you'd be a lot healthier.

SS: You mentioned previously a list of diseases caused by anaerobic cell reproduction. Do you have CanCell programmed to different frequencies for different diseases?

ES: No, I establish 34 energy clusters so it has a whole family of frequencies in it. See this is one of the problems with the FDA, because they think things happen chemically and all allopathic drags work vibrationally. Nothing works chemically.

See, you can go back to the later works of Einstein and he's telling the same thing I'm telling you in different words. He admits that there exists nothing in the universe except electromagnetic vibrational frequency. There is no such thing as mass. There is no particle in the nucleus of the atom. These things just simply don't exist. The only thing that exists is various forms of vibrational densities that appear to our perceptions as mass or solids.

SS: Is CanCell legal to use?

ES: It is not legal. Actually, it is legal but the US Government is using the full power of the government to prohibit people from exercising their first amendment right to freedom of speech or freedom of choice. They have unlawfully, without jurisdiction, prohibited me from giving this to people. Before the government felt they didn't want the competition from something that was effective, people would call me on the phone or write and inform me that they were diagnosed with terminal cancer. At that point I would send them CanCell with instructions and diet. If they followed the routine, about 8 out of 10 people ended up without cancer.

SS: How many people received CanCell?

ES: I've given away well over 30,000 treatments. Our files probably have about 10,000 testimonial letters, many complete with medical records. The dosage would be 1/2 cc under the tongue and 1/2 cc at a pulse point on the body.

SS: How much did it cost?

ES: I have never charged for it. I made a gift of this to everyone who needed help and I even paid for postage. There was no money involved and I sent back all donations.

SS: So if the FDA could conclude that CanCell was simply water, how could they block its use?

ES: In the hearing, Judge Bernard Friedman declared that water was a drug on the record. Secondly, when the Keyfaver Amendment FDA Act of 1938 came in in 1962, the 1962 amendment grandfathered all drugs that were in the market-place prior to 1938, then CanCell should be grandfathered in. I filed a motion which he ignored. So I will resubmit that motion sometime this week.

Today, there is an unlawful injunction in place and they have prevented me from making a gift of this to anyone.

Back in 1990, the National Cancer Institute asked me for a sample of CanCell. We sent it to them. They tested it on 58 different tumour strains. It reduced or eliminated all 58. It was 100% effective. They put this in a report and signed it. They're sorry they signed it because now they are denying they ever did the study. They're trying their best not to let people know that there is something that would be helpful.

A little later, we were doing double-blind studies under World Health and FDA protocols on the AIDS virus in Africa. We were getting computer analyses of the data that we generated at the Texas Medical Center. They published an article in the *Explore!* magazine in July 1992. It said the people who were on CanCell with an additive to it had an increase in the CD4 count of their immune system of 604 points, and the placebo group had a decrease of 102 points. That upset them because that of course is the next great boondoggle in the world: how much money can we spend on AIDS research? So once they found out that you cannot get an increase of that magnitude in the CD4 count if the virus is still there, the conclusion was of course that CanCell is an effective treatment for AIDS. We know it is. We've done over 1000 double-blind studies in Africa and to this date the people who are doing the studies have refused to give me the studies of the report. The last reports, as I understand, were filed by the World Health Organisation.

So they do know. The data is there. The US Government tested it and know it works and that is the reason they are so upset.

SS: So what's your next step?

ES: Well, we're fighting it. I would prefer to have the government follow the law. Once you get into law and this lawsuit that was brought against me, the first thing you have to understand is federal statutes. These federal statutes that you and I are subjected to apply only to corporate entities and to individuals who have signed a contract with the federal government. They admitted in open court that they do not have a contract with me and therefore, technically, they do not have jurisdiction over me or over CanCell. But they went ahead with the case.

The second point in this case is that they proceeded without a plaintiff. There was no harmed party. The FDA actually went out and tried to solicit a harmed party. They got names of people I sent CanCell to through the United Parcel Service, which was unlawful, but they did it. They went out and interviewed these people and none of them would sign or testify against me. Almost every one of them said that they would testify on my behalf.

So because there was no harmed party, there was never a hearing. I have the right to face my accuser. There wasn't an accuser. So Judge Friedman broke the law when he issued a permanent injunction prohibiting me from making a gift of CanCell to anyone. His law says that he must issue a temporary injunction to determine if it does irreparable harm. Obviously it doesn't. He issued a permanent injunction. When I put a motion in to set it aside on the basis that it was unlawful, he put in writing that since I was giving it away, of course it didn't do me any harm. The only people it harmed were those individuals who were benefiting from taking CanCell. So he admitted that. My reaction to all of this was that I continued to give CanCell because he did not enjoin me from making a gift of CanCell. The original injunction said he enjoined me from shipping a drug in interstate commerce. Of course commerce is what you do for a profit. So I kept giving it to people, but when I gave it to them I asked them to send a copy of their medical records to Judge Friedman, so he knew that he had erred by putting this injunction in place.

Friedman admitted in the show cause hearing that he had an extensive file that indicates that CanCell cures many different diseases and therefore it must be a drug.

When I appealed the original decision, they said I could not appeal it because I had to have a transcript before I could appeal it Since there was never a hearing there was no transcript. When I tried to point that out, Judge Friedman perjured himself on the record in writing over a 7-month period telling that there was a transcript, it was lost, it was in transit, it was misplaced etc. When I tried to appeal the entire case, the appeals court came back to me twice and said that they do not have jurisdiction over the case.

So it is at a standstill and it's obvious that it has to be a conspiracy since you have involved in this the FDA, the AMA and the American Cancer Society. You have Judge Friedman knowingly breaking the law and the appeals court knowingly has jurisdiction but says that they don't. When you get all of this together, it's obvious that there is a conspiracy to prevent the people from being able to use something that would benefit them.

I always thought that this was close to genocide. The International AIDS Foundation has filed a lawsuit in the international courts in Europe charging the US Government with bioethics violation, and it was accepted several weeks ago. This suit has to do with AZT, not CanCell. We'll see how that proceeds. If enough people scream, it will move. If not, they will bury it.

SS: How does CanCell work on AIDS?

ES: The same as the Memorex commercial on TV works. It hits the interference pattern that causes the virus to disassociate, to break up. It is quite effective. Our data indicates in 21 days it is 98% effective and that's actually reading the virus in the blood, not looking at CD4 counts. We actually put blood samples on a microscope, use a fluorescent dye and then read the virus in the blood. The original double-blind study had 101 people on CanCell and of that 101 people, 99 people were virus-free.

SS: Does CanCell work on all viruses and pathogens?

ES: Oh yes. Over in Africa instead of coming down with Kaposi's or something else, most of them came down with viral meningitis. The researchers in Africa tell me that CanCell knocks off viral meningitis in 4 days.

There is no such thing as an incurable disease any longer.

The only thing is that we just simply have not been able to apply or know what to apply to those diseases to get rid of them. CanCell is what I consider one of those advances in technology pointing to the point that nothing is incurable.

SS: So the body at optimum health has a certain frequency. If you have something that is going to help the body to eliminate various diseases with various characteristics, it must be helping the body to reestablish its own health frequency. So it matters not what the disease is; the body is out of tune with itself, and all you are doing with CanCell is reminding it of its natural frequency and the body gravitates toward it. Then anything in the way of that harmony would be dissipated.

ES: That's pretty good. Yes. You know, several years ago we had about 35 to 40 people in the Seattle area taking CanCell for AIDS and they were all responding. They were working through the University of Washington. Then all of a sudden something happened and it all folded within a couple of weeks. There are a lot of people in that area that had taken CanCell successfully for AIDS.

One of the problems I have with the younger generation who have AIDS and take CanCell: they gain weight and the T4 cells go up and back to normal, then 6 months later I get a call and they say they need another bottle—they got it again. I say, "You haven't learned anything and changed your lifestyle?" "Well no, why should I? The material is free and it's easy to get rid of so why should I change?" Whatever people are doing to expose themselves to the AIDS virus, don't do it!

Also, we do know that only 29% of those people who are exposed to the AIDS virus that become HIV-positive ever come down with AIDS. The immune system can control the virus and does control the virus in the majority of the cases. It's debatable once someone is exposed how long it is until they can show symptoms. They can remain normal and still be HIV-positive unless they get into a stressful situation or their health is damaged. That could dump their immune system, then they could become symptomatic.

We are spending $4.9 billion tax dollars researching AIDS. Of course you have to understand that the purpose of research is to accumulate knowledge, not to find a cure for AIDS.

SS: So the question is, how is CanCell made?

ES: About a year ago I was at the Texas Medical Center with a Dr Arthur Erikson. We were discussing the effects of CanCell on the AIDS virus. After about 3 days of meetings I got up and said to the group that CanCell is so far advanced beyond medical technology that there is not even a vocabulary in place that we can use to explain it to the medical scientists. Our first order of business is to develop a vocabulary.

So it's hard to tell people how you deprogramme and programme water. It does have memory. However, no mechanical device touches it, no electricity. It's all done differently. If you had the vibrational frequency of the 60-cycle current, that would destroy it. If you used magnets or any metallic device, that also has a vibrational frequency and those frequencies would tend to override.

SS: Could you give us a hint? Is it done through human consciousness?

ES: Only partly. That does have an effect upon it. The human mind can destroy it. Not only mine but anyone else's. This IS part of positive thinking. I don't know how spiritually inclined you are, but one of my observations goes like this: it is the intent that the individual who is creating the material,

70

their mental intent has an effect upon the product. The reason conventional or allopathic medicine doesn't work and never will work is because those individuals that are creating it are creating it not to cure anybody, but their main intent is to make a profit. It does make the profit but it is not effective as a cure. So you would have to change the entire effort of the medical profession and the pharmaceutical industry before you could get allopathic medicines to work again. I don't care what Clinton does or anyone else, unless they make some basic change there, nothing they do is going to work, unfortunately.

If you read a couple of hundred books on the art of positive thinking and that type of subject material, well then you will start to change the direction that you are thinking and you'll be right where you should be. Try not to be too scientific about it. Every time someone does they get it all screwed up.

This material is advanced to the point where you have to go back and start with Einstein and realise that he in his later writings indicated that nothing exists in the universe except electromagnetic vibrational frequency. There is no such thing as mass. Once you understand that and that everything is electrovibrational magnetic energy, then everything else becomes quite plain. Again, what we consider mass or solids are simply vibrational densities. If you can agree with that, then the rest of all of this becomes easy, because all you're doing is providing a vibrational catalyst that allows the body to tune itself or become in vibrational balance. When it does that it eliminates all vibrational density in the body. When it eliminates the vibrational density which we call disease, the disease no longer exists. That's purely and simply all it is.

SS: So couldn't a person who is clear in their attitude and consciousness infuse those vibrations into a substance which could carry that vibration?

ES: Yes, you can do that. But at the same time, if you can do that you could cure any illness you had. The mind is powerful enough to do that. This is what they call the placebo effect. The placebo effect actually runs close to 30% in many cases.

SS: So CanCell is more that just someone holding up a bottle of water and thinking into it.

ES: Oh absolutely. Yes.

SS: It's a whole new non-technical field of technology.

Part 2: How Our Healing Water Works

About 20 years ago scientists discovered that water molecules could store memory. Dr. Masaru Emoto achieved fame with his New York Time's bestseller book "The Hidden Messages In Water." He showed that the molecular structure of water changed with the type of memory placed into the water, and he developed methods of photography to show molecules of water after being imprinted with various types of positive and negative messages. IBM scientists, as we speak, are researching ways to harness the memory storage ability of water molecules in order to develop better computer memory storage capacity.

All water carries the memories and information that have been implanted into it. Some of our water has been around for thousands of years. Therefore it carries memory imprints of its experiences during these thousands of years. Some of these memories were positive (the joy of a childbirth, for example) and some of these memories were negative (the massacre of an Indian village, for example).

Your body is 80 to 90 percent water. You know this. What you did not realize is that the water in the cells of your body still carries all of its previous memory, some of which is positive, some of which is negative. That is okay, as your body is used to dealing with this situation.

About 15 years ago a researcher named Ed Sopcak interviewed approximately 100 people who had cancer. Without exception, he found that all of these people had suffered a severe negative experience from six months to twenty-four months prior to the onset of their cancer. Examples of these negative experiences were divorce, termination of employment, betrayal by a spouse or friend, or loss of a child or loved one. Based on this interesting information, Mr. Sopcak developed the postulation that the cancer cell was based on a negative frequency vibration. He experimented. He was an electrical engineer, so he used an electrical approach to solving his problem. He was quite successful, and for a number of years he cured thousands of cases of cancer. Here is how he did it:

1. He used principles of electrical engineering to remove all previous memory from some water.
2. He then subjected the water to only positive memories (mostly the vibrations of love and harmony).

3. Then he fed this only-positive vibration water to his people who had cancer. Their cancer went away.
4. Mr. Sopcak explains what happens as follows: "When the water that has only positive vibrations in it is taken into the body, it is foreign to all of the water in your body that is comprised of both positive and negative vibrations. It is especially foreign to the cancer cells that are made up of only negative vibrations. These cancer molecules, made up of only negative vibrations, are thrown into disarray by the arrival on the scene of molecules of water that are all positive. This disrupts the frequency patterns of the negative-only cancer cells, allowing your body's natural defense and immune system to remove them and expel them from the body."
5. Mr. Sopcak then later discovered that these same healing principles applied to many other of the body's illness and diseases.

In approximately 1990 Ed Sopcak appeared on the nationwide Maury Popich television show, explaining his method and introducing many people who had been cured of their cancer using his water. He named his water Cancell. Unfortunately Mr. Sopcak dies shortly thereafter, and his healing system has never been further developed.

In 2002 Dr. Masaru Emoto basically rediscovered this healing modality. He uses a different method to remove the memory from the water (he uses distillation) and then instills the water with only loving positive memories. He has named his healing water "Hado Water". His method is explained in his books, which are available on amazon.com.

Part 3: How to Make and Install a Healing Water Device on your home's water pipes:

What You Need

A. The demagnetizer strip

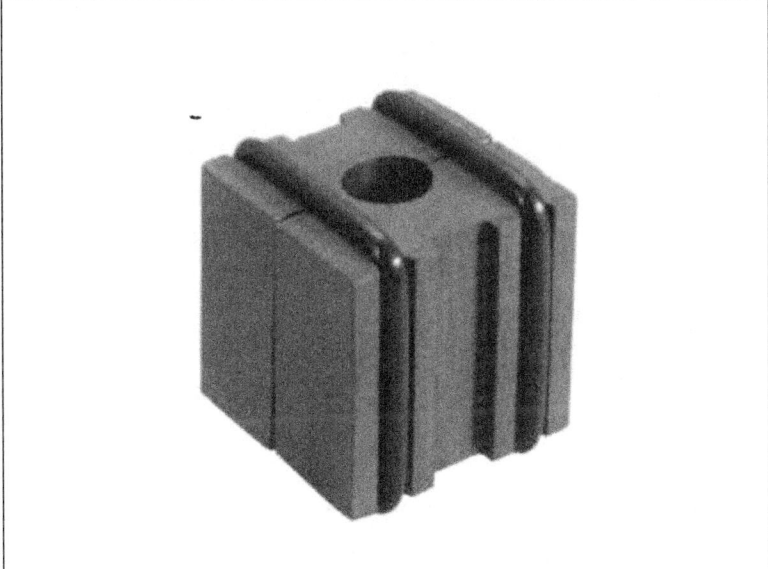

General Tool 360 Demagnetizer. It takes 6 of these to make a demagnetizer strip

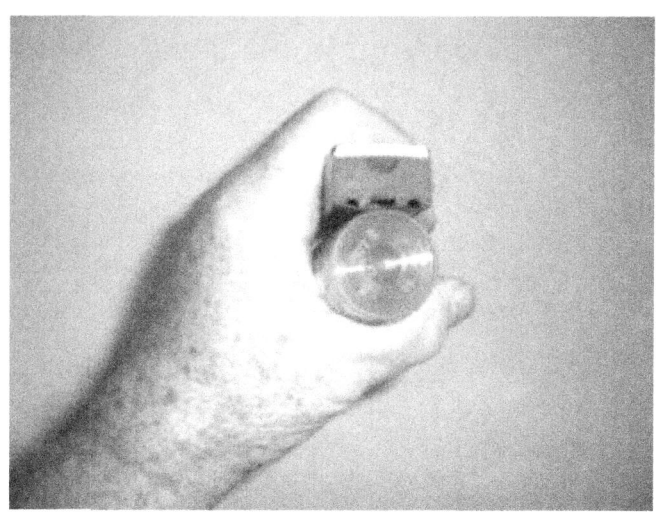

End view of 12 inch demagnetizer strip showing its placement on a water pipe. Note that the oval channel of the magnetizers is placed away from the pipe. Very important.

Please note above (right) that 12 demagnetizer magnets are taped to a 12 inch paint stirrer stick as shown. The placement of the magnets on the stick, and the subsequent placement of the demagnetizer stick on the pipe must be correct. Keep the oval channel of the magnets away from the pipe.

You will need the following:

    a. Six General Tool 360 Demagnitizers. You can buy them on the internet or go to http://www.generaltool.com. They cost $3.18 each.

    b. A roll of regular black electrical tape (3/4 in wide).

c. A thin wooden strip, 1/8 to ¼ inch in thickness and 1 in by 12 inches. For this I get a free paint stirrer at the paint section of WalMart. It is the perfect size.

Do the following:

a. Strip the rubber bands from the magnetizers and separate the 12 separate magnet units.
b. Tape the units to the stick as shown. You will now have a demagnetizer strip that is 1 ft. long.
c. Tape or tie this unit to the water pipe in your home. Place it 3 ft. ahead of the energy card/plate.
d. Be sure to have the side of the demagnetizers with the large oval away from the pipe.
e. Note: Keep this demagnetizer strip at least 3 ft. away from your energy card at all times. Otherwise you may damage the energy card.

B. The energizer plate

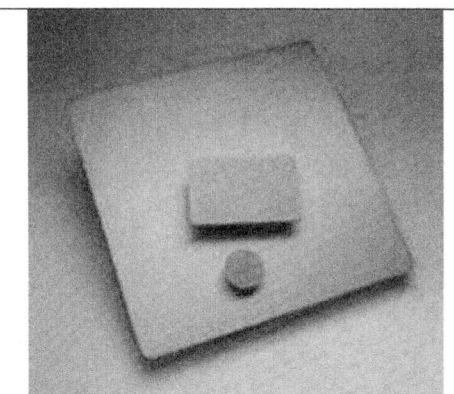

Use the small energy plate that is approximately 2 ¾ " by 4 ½" in size.

You can find a suitable energy plate at http://www.energyplates.com/plates.html. Order the "small" plate. They cost about $15.00.

Tape the plate on the water pipe 3 ft. downstream of the demagnetizer strip.

Comments on Healing Water Device Hookup

Basic principle: First discovered by Ed Sopcak in the 1980's, and later rediscovered by Dr. Masaru Emoto several years ago (as elaborated upon in his best-seller book *The Hidden Messages in Water*), we perform the following:

1. First the water is passed by a demagnetizer. This removes all memory from the molecules of water.
2. Then the demagnetized (dememorized) water is passed by an energizer, which places only positive vibrations into the water. The best healing energies are *Love and Gratitude*.

Points to watch out for:

1. Locate a section of water pipe entering the house. Usually this will be ¾ in. or ½ in. copper or PVC pipe.
2. Fasten the demagnetizer strip and the energizer plate onto the pipe, placing them at least three ft. apart. This is so the demagnetizer does not interfere with

the energizer plate (which has positive energizers magnetically embedded in it). Be sure that the demagnetizer strip is placed first so that the water flows past the demagnetizer strip before it reaches the energizer plate.

3. You may use tape or plastic electrical ties to fasten the demagnetizer strip and the energizer plate/card to the pipe. I use black electrical tape.

4. Sometimes, because of the layout of the pipe in your house, you are not able to separate the demagnetizer strip and the plate by at least 3 ft.. In this case, place them as far apart as is possible. Then wrap the energizer plate and the pipe to which it is attached with at least 4 layers of aluminum foil. This will help to shield the energy plate from any stray demagnetic effects of the demagnetizer strip. In no case get the aluminum foil between the plate/card and the pipe to which it is attached because this would interfere with the energizer plate passing its positive vibrations to the water passing through the pipe.

5. If it is necessary to install the healing device under your kitchen sink, it may not be possible to keep the demagnetizer strip and the energizer plate 3 ft. apart. In this case, place the plate as close to the faucet as possible. Then wrap the energizer plate and the pipe to which it is attached with 4 layers of aluminum foil. This should adequately protect the plate from being demagnetized (ruined). Then install the demagnetizer strip as far from the plate as possible. It is best to attach the system to the cold water pipe.

6. As far as I know, this mechanism never wears out.

Final Comments:

The total cost of treating the everyday water that I drink is almost nothing. I fill old 1.5 liter wine bottles with water and place them in the sacred geometry 3-tubes, and process them for 3 days in my kitchen pantry. The only real cost is for the mailing tube sections that I use to make the cylinders that I keep in my kitchen pantry. They will last a lifetime.

The cost of making and installing a healing water device on my home water pipes was less than $100. It will also last a lifetime.

I love a bargain. These two systems for making structured water are bargains!

In addition, for approximately $300 you can find and install on your water pipes a system that imparts a Viktor Shauberger "spin" to your drinking water. Search the Internet for these devices.

I also order the herbal tea at http://www.remedies.net that is made with structured water. I get my immune system bolstered by the tea, and get their structured water as a bonus.

With these gadgets and features added to your inventory, you and your family are in for a delightful treat. Now just try to explain all this to your friends. Lots of luck!

Bibliography

Laurence Gardner, *Lost Secrets of the sacred Ark*, ISBN 0-767-7598-2

Robert E. Cox, *the Elixir of Immortality*, ISBN 978-159477303-7

Chris Emmons, *Ormus Modern Day Alchemy*, ISBN 978-0-9815840-1-0

Henry Kroll, *The Philosopher Stone; Immortality Discovered* ISBN 1-932672-24-9

R.A. Schwaller de Lubicz, *Sacred Science*, ISBN 0-89281-222-2

A Treatise: How Ormus repairs DNA and how it works

This information in this section is extracted from the book *The Philosopher Stone* by Henry Kroll.

In order for body cells to replicate they have to split the genes of the old cell to produce a new cell, the old cell sharing the genes with the new cell. The process of "unzipping" the gene codes completely, without damaging the gene codes, requires that certain minerals be present. These minerals are the monatomic mineral state of gold and platinum.

This critical process is made more difficult in these modern times because of our mineral-deficient diets. The soils that most of our vegetables and fruits are grown on have long-ago become deficient in most of the 84 minerals and trace elements that we need for perfect health. Linus Pauling, two-time Nobel Prize winner, stated, "You can trace every sickness, every disease and every ailment to a mineral deficiency".

Each time a cell replicates, it loses a few of the gene chains called tellimires. When enough of the tellimires are gone, the cell dies. Thus it is the loss of these tellimires in the body cells that causes aging. If a cell has enough of the right superconducting minerals during cell replication it doesn't lose any tellimires. Therefore it can replicate indefinitely.

If a person's body is saturated with monatomic-state elements of gold and platinum, it is possible for a person to live for hundreds of years free of disease and without the problems of aging. [Perhaps this helps to explain the Old Testament people who were reported to live for many hundreds of years.]

In addition, the monatomic-state silver minerals in Ormus also play an important part in your health. The monatomic silver elements are tied to the very process of life itself. Monatomic silver kills disease organisms, promotes major growth of bone, and accelerates the healing of body tissue. It also speeds up the cell replication process.

Concerning the type of people who are able to accept ormus into their lives, Mr. Kroll states, "Some people are drawn into this knowledge from a very deep part of their soul". Enough said. If you are reading this, this probably means you.

Moses had several methods of making manna. When they were travelling in the desert, he and his brother Aaron took desert soil that was high in alkalinity and boiled it in alkaline water for several days. As the water boiled away, they added more alkaline water that they got from certain desert springs, making the brew even more alkaline. They then cooled the high-alkaline mixture and added vinegar to drop the ph. As the ph dropped, a milky substance formed. This was the monatomic states of the precious metals previously mentioned. The clear liquid was poured off, and the milky substance that was left over was their manna. This milky liquid was baked into whatever grains they had with them, and the resulting loaves were their "shewbread", their life-sustaining food that got them through the desert wilderness.

Anyone who has made Ormus using the Wet Method will be impressed with the similarities between these two methods.

Our Amazing Healing Discovery

In 2021 I made my most important healing discovery. I wish to share it with you. So here goes.

I began to study artificial intelligence. In reading up on the QFS (quantum financial system) that was just beginning to emerge in the banking system, I found some intriguing and hard-to-believe information. There was plenty of information available about what the QFS would do for mankind (better, faster banking, more honest and dependable system, etc.) there was little or no information about how it worked.

I have a personal rule; if I don't understand it, I avoid it. So I jumped into a quick study to see if I could understand it, since it seemed so important to the future of mankind.

Briefly, what I discovered is that as computers got more and more sophisticated, and faster and faster, and more "intelligent", scientists were reaching the point where they had learned how to interface computers with the human mind. I will not go any further in this explanation, because, frankly, it get freaky and hard-to-believe if you go any deeper.

As I was working my way through all of this, I got some advice in meditation. My spirit guides advised me not to fret because mankind had already been using this technology for a thousand years. They then mentioned the Holy Water used by the Catholic Church.

Years ago, when I practiced Radionics healing extensively, I had, yes, learned that Holy Water does have special healing power. I had actually bought some Holy Water online, placed it in test tube, and had used it as a "reagent" to speed up certain healing processes. In other words, when I added the vibrational qualities of the Holy Water to the vibrations that were being sent to a person's affliction, the healing process was improved. So I knew that Holy Water was special.

I next went to the Internet to learn more about Holy water. Here is how it is made; a group of Priests fill a church fountain or other container with water and then they pray over it. They, in essence, bless the water. Then it becomes Holy Water. Pretty simple.

There are 3 prayers that they may use for this process. All are basically the same. Here is one of them:

"Blessed are you, Lord, all-powerful God, who in Christ, the living water of salvation, blessed and transformed us. Grant that when we are sprinkled with this water or make use of it, we will be refreshed inwardly by the power of the Holy Spirit and continue to walk in the new life we received at Baptism."

I was surprised that the simplicity of this prayer. Basically, all it does is commit the water to the wonderful power of God.

Then things got really wonderful and special. This is hard to explain, but I will try my best to explain it to you.

I was told that the water being blessed and prayed over was capable of assisting mankind much more. But it had to be instructed by God to do so. Then the water would directly (in the case of illness), attack and remove the illness. Or in case of emotional distress, remove the harmful emotions and restore the body to happiness and balance.

Basically, this process changes the water in your body from a passive status to a status where it becomes an active healing agent. It was emphatically stressed that, unless the water as asked by God to do this, it would not work.

Where an understanding of Artificial Intelligence comes in

If you ponder on this for a while, as I have done, things become more clear. Artificial Intelligence involves establishing a link with the human mind and a non-human object (the computer). This link goes through God. God somehow allows this link (information) to be passed on to other mechanisms in God's realm, and the work is done. Not a great explanation, but is the best that I can offer, given my own limitations.

Well, the same basic thing happens with Holy Water. I have explained this in other sections of my book "On Stormy Seas". The written works of Viktor Shauberger and Masaru Emoto delve sufficiently into water's ability to carry conscience and intelligence.

Thus when the Priests pray over the water, they impart a request that God bless the water with their message. God does this, and from then on the water has special curative powers. The water then later passes this curative power on to you.

So my Spirit Guides are right. The enlightenment of our knowledge of artificial intelligence does lead us right back to the knowledge of Holy Water that has been known for a thousand years. Interesting.

Where are we going with this?

I have to be careful here, as I do not wish to inadvertently reveal anything that I am not supposed to reveal.

What my Spiritual Advisors have told me is to take the basic prayer to bless Holy Water and "soup" it up by asking the water to do extra things, which it will most probably be happy to do for you and God. Remember always that God is approving everything, so you cannot inadvertently ask for anything that goes against God's will. Should you accidently do so, it is simple. God will not grant your request.

So, my first chance to use this knowledge came when two of my beloved Essiac employees got sick from taking Covid vaccinations shots. They drank this water. They immediately got better. I have also been using this knowledge to improve my own health and well as helping my wife deal with some health issues. It is working for us.

I am going to list here several of the requests that we have been using.

Dear God, Please instruct this water to remove all harmful substances from my body. Please remove all illness and disease from my body. Please remove all harm from the Covid and the Covid vaccinations. Thank you. We love you.	**Dear God, Please instruct the water in my body to restore my energy levels to that of a 35 year-old person. Thank you and I love you.**

Dear God, Please instruct this water to heal And cure the swelling in my feet And legs. Thank you. I love you.	Dear God, Please instruct this water to remove the excess and unhealthy fat from my body And restore my body shape to a healthy Condition. I love you. Thank you.

Using Energy Plates to assist us

Here is the system that I use; I use a credit card sized energy plate. I buy mine at purpleplates.com. These aluminum plates are imbued with life force energy. I have used them successfully for many years for other healing purposes. I then perform a consecration ritual where I pass the message for my healing to the energy plate, all the while asking God to approve everything. I then print the prayer request, cut it out, ask God to bless it (through a prayer) and tape it to the energy plate. I cover everything in plastic. I then take this energy plate and tape it or fasten it to the water pipe feeding the faucet where I draw my drinking and cooking water. Sometimes, depending on the complexity of the house water piping system, I just fasten the plate to the cold water line that feeds the house (usually near the water heater).

Thus the blessed message is passed on to the water that I drink. The water does the rest. Some people prefer to carry the energy plate in their pocket. Either method works.

After a while you may get your own inspiration on various ways to use this information. Just be sure to get God's permission.

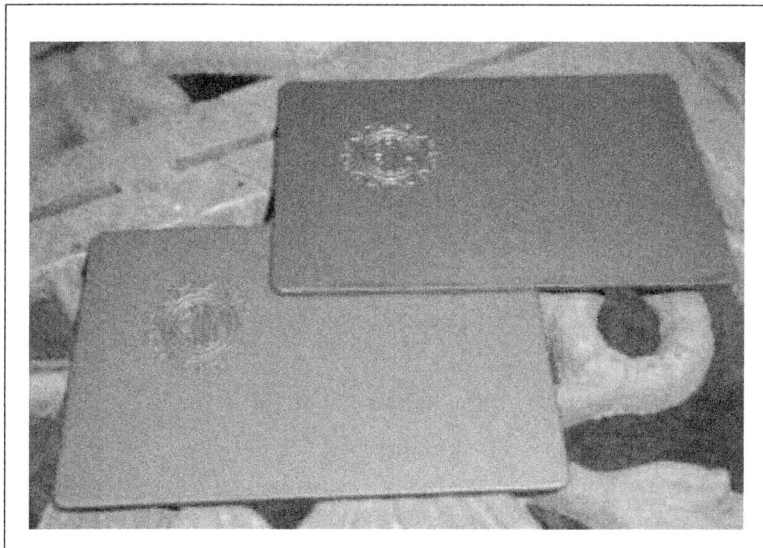

Energy plates (credit card size)

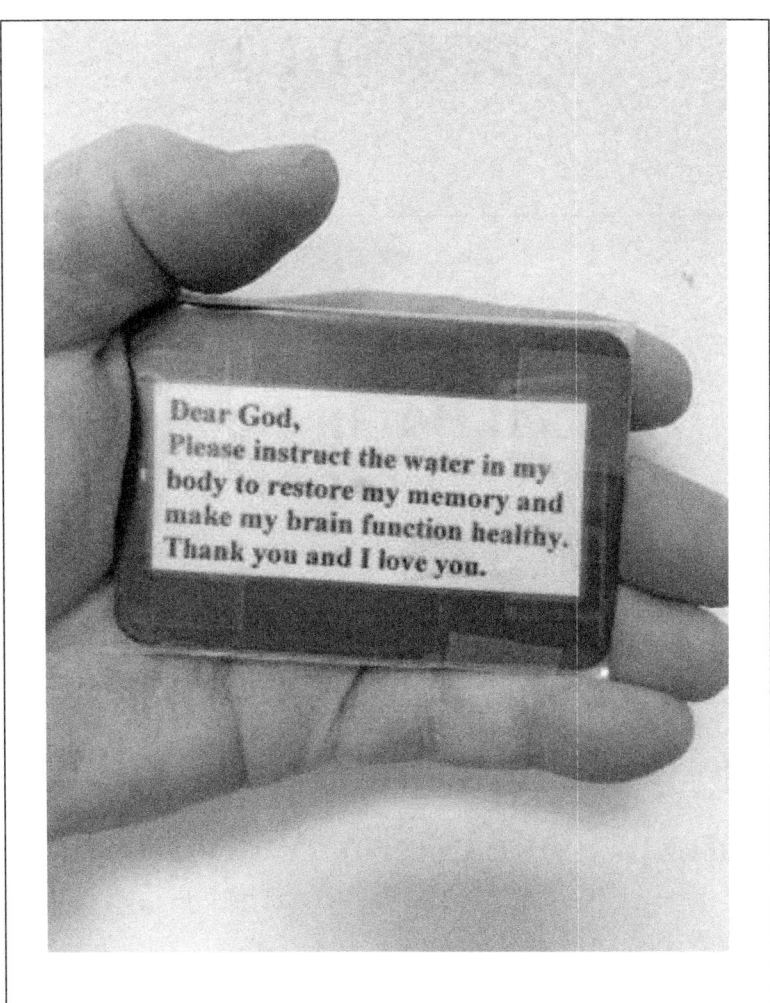

The finished product

ADDENDUM

Special Bonus Section

Do you know anyone who has skin cancer? If so, you may wish to show them this information. This inexpensive cream really works!

Our "Super Dooper Skin Cancer Salve"

There are two ingredients in our Super Dooper akin cancer salve:

Hydrogen Peroxide.

The main ingredient is liquid hydrogen peroxide. It is not just any-old drug store variety of peroxide. It is a special kind of hydrogen peroxide that is labeled **"35% Food Grade Hydrogen Peroxide"**.

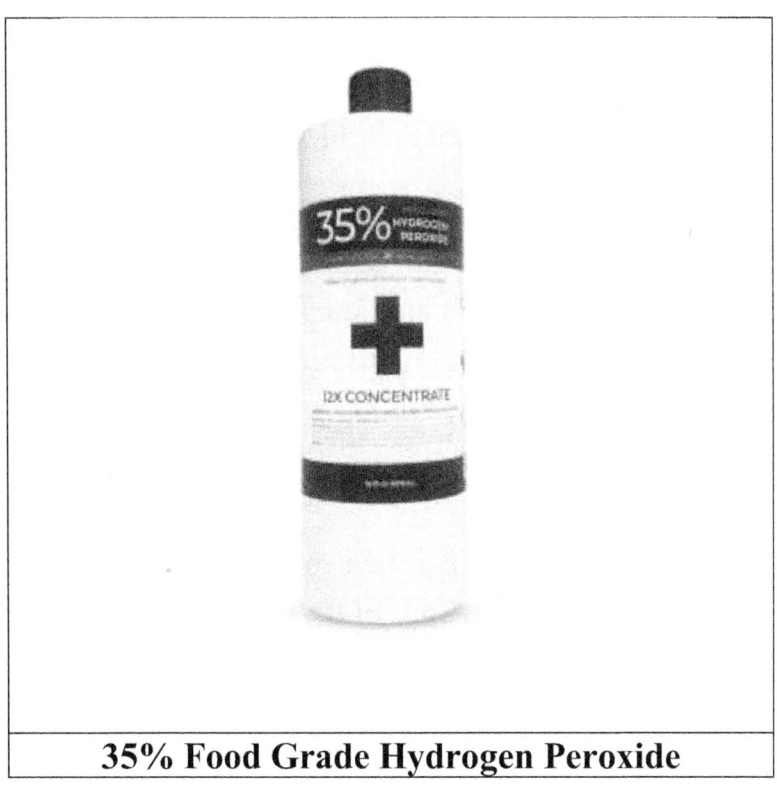

35% Food Grade Hydrogen Peroxide

This special peroxide can be found at many health food stores, or it can be bought online.

The last 16 oz. bottle that I bought cost me about $20.00. It will last me about 6 months.

How it works.

The chemical expression for hydrogen peroxide is H_2O_2. When the hydrogen peroxide is placed on your skin, it transfers to H_2O (water) and O (a free molecule of oxygen). This free molecule of oxygen is very reactive. It wants to quickly bond with something else.

If the hydrogen peroxide has been placed on a malignant tumor (such as a skin cancer tumor) it will quickly bond with the tumor.

But the cancerous tumor is anaerobic; it cannot exist in the presence of oxygen. Thus it immediately dies.

And that, dear friend is how it works. It works fast. It is simple to apply. And, in my many years of using this salve, I have never failed to see it work properly.

A few words of caution.

Hydrogen peroxide is very sensitive to light. If it is not stored in a dark place, it will deteriorate quickly. It should be kept is a light- proof bottle, and the bottle should be stored in a cool, dark place.

Also, it should be replaced every year-or-so. Age will reduce its strength.

Aloe Vera Gel.

The other ingredient is aloe vera gel.

This is easier to obtain. You can find it at almost any drug store, grocery store, or health food store. A 16 oz. bottle or jar costs me about $16.00.

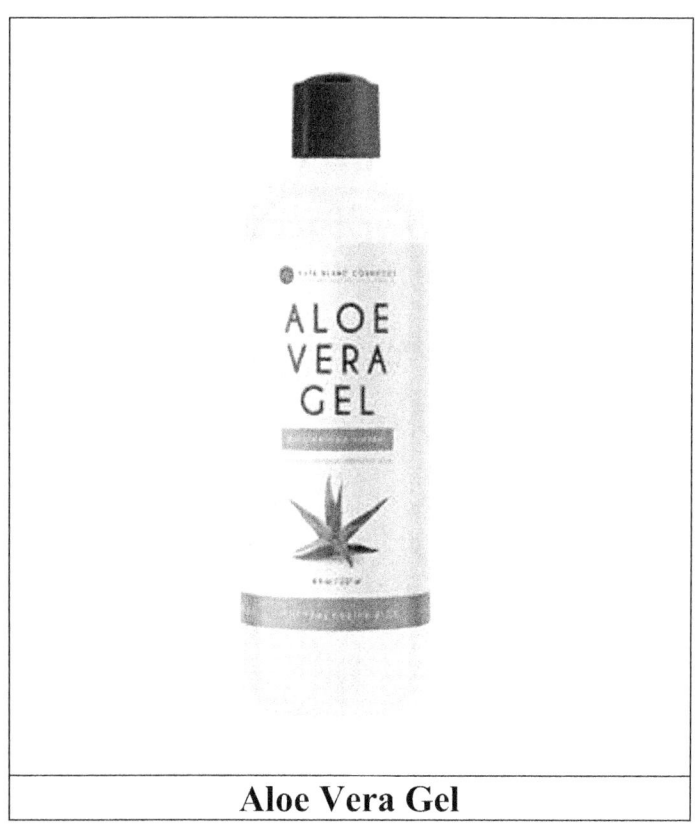

Aloe Vera Gel

Making the Salve:

Making the salve is incredibly easy. Just mix up the amount that you will need. Make the ration about 50% peroxide and 50% aloe vera gel. It is that simple.

You may want to use a plastic, wood or metal spoon for your mixing, as the 35% peroxide is very strong and may burn your fingers.

Store your salve in a light-proof bottle and keep in in a dark place (a refrigerator works fine).

Using the Salve:

Apply the salve to your skin cancer as needed. The more you apply, the faster it will act.

If, when you apply the salve, you see a bubbling action, this is a really good sign. The bubbling action is the active oxygen molecule in the peroxide mixing with the cancerous growth.

You should see results within a few days.

Note: This information is extracted from the book **"The Skin Cancer Information Handbook"** by Michael D. Miller.

Another Bonus Section!

Let's have some fun! By reading this book, you have shown that you are an open-minded person. So I now wish to offer you the following information.

Pyramid Power

How to shave for almost free!

My dad was an interesting guy. Raised on a farm in Minnesota during the Depression, he didn't have an opportunity to get an education. But he was smart, and had an inquiring mind. He read a lot.

So back in the 1970's he sent me a book titled "Pyramid Power". Interesting book, it elaborated on the special powers of a pyramid built with the geometric ratios of the Great Pyramid of Egypt. In the book, it stated that if you placed a shaving razor at a point 1/3 down from the apex of the pyramid, that the razor would stay sharp.

Many years later, I remembered this. So when I was experimenting with some small replicas of the Great

Pyramid, I tried this experiment. It worked. For years I kept my shaving razor sharp with this method. But it was awkward because of the difficulty in keeping a pyramid structure in the vicinity of my bathroom. The smallest pyramid that I could fine to use was about 24 inches wide and 19 inches tall. There was never enough space in my bathroom to use the device. So I gradually stopped using it.

Here is what I learned: I could use an ordinary disposable razor. Normally such a razor would stay sharp for about a week, then had to be thrown away. I could place it under the apex of the pyramid. And then it lasted me for up to six months. Pretty neat. But as I mentioned, it was very inconvenient to use because of the bulky size of the pyramid.

Well friends, I have just made another discovery that I wish to share with you. I have found a very small brass pyramid that works well to keep my razor sharp. The brass pyramid is only 2 inches square, so it fits on my bathroom shelf nicely. And I bought it on the Internet for less than $10.00. I placed my razor (shown in the picture) on the apex of the pyramid as shown. I started using this disposable razor in January of this year. It is now

August, and the razor is a sharp as it was on the first day I used it (maybe even sharper).

Here is a picture of my rig:

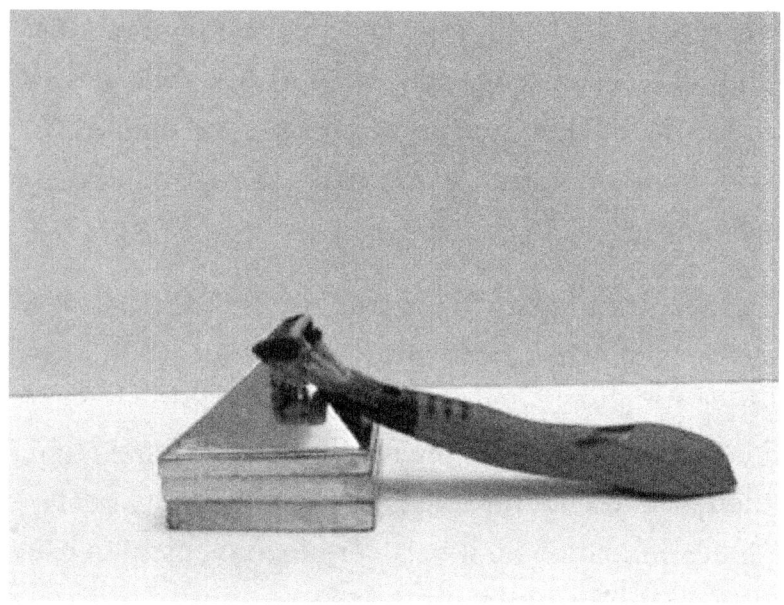

In case any of you wish to experiment with this rig, you can google "small brass pyramid". Mine came as a set of 3 pyramids. I stacked them as shown in the photo for maximum power.

As I mentioned before, the set of 3 small brass pyramids cost me around $10.00. Then the razor cost me about $3.00. If they last for a year, my total cost of shaving for the year will be $13.00. Not bad! And I still have the pyramids!

By the way, here is a list of books that I have written (some with pen names). They are available on amazon.com.

On Stormy Seas	Elk Hunting Guide
Increasing Your Cat's Life & Longevity	Kill Zone
Increasing Your Dog's Longevity	Egyptian Sacred Geometry
The Lyme Disease Handbook	Pirate History of Florida
Women's Beauty Secrets	Essiac Story and 6 Examples
Defending Against the Ambush	Two Essiac Angels
The Diabetes Handbook	Essiac Handbook
Salt and Your Health	Essiac Testimonials
Structured Water for Greater Health and Happiness	A Terrible Beauty
Greater Longevity; Rediscovering the Philosopher's Stone	Sacred Geometry Healing Water
Healing Water and Cancer	Male Menopause
	Women's Health Secrets
	Beating Arthritis
	Douglas MacArthur; from Betrayal to Victory

Printed in Great Britain
by Amazon

22506183R00056